PHTHALATES
AND CUMULATIVE
RISK ASSESSMENT

The Tasks Ahead

Committee on the Health Risks of Phthalates

Board on Environmental Studies and Toxicology

Division on Earth and Life Studies

NATIONAL RESEARCH COUNCIL
OF THE NATIONAL ACADEMIES

THE NATIONAL ACADEMIES PRESS
Washington, D.C.
www.nap.edu

THE NATIONAL ACADEMIES PRESS   **500 Fifth Street, NW**   **Washington, DC 20001**

NOTICE: The project that is the subject of this report was approved by the Governing Board of the National Research Council, whose members are drawn from the councils of the National Academy of Sciences, the National Academy of Engineering, and the Institute of Medicine. The members of the committee responsible for the report were chosen for their special competences and with regard for appropriate balance.

This project was supported by Contract 68-C-03-081 between the National Academy of Sciences and the U.S. Environmental Protection Agency. Any opinions, findings, conclusions, or recommendations expressed in this publication are those of the authors and do not necessarily reflect the view of the organizations or agencies that provided support for this project.

International Standard Book Number-13: 978-0-309-12841-4
International Standard Book Number-10: 0-309-12841-2

Additional copies of this report are available from:

The National Academies Press
500 Fifth Street, NW
Box 285
Washington, DC 20055

800-624-6242
202-334-3313 (in the Washington metropolitan area)
http://www.nap.edu

THE NATIONAL ACADEMIES
Advisers to the Nation on Science, Engineering, and Medicine

The **National Academy of Sciences** is a private, nonprofit, self-perpetuating society of distinguished scholars engaged in scientific and engineering research, dedicated to the furtherance of science and technology and to their use for the general welfare. Upon the authority of the charter granted to it by the Congress in 1863, the Academy has a mandate that requires it to advise the federal government on scientific and technical matters. Dr. Ralph J. Cicerone is president of the National Academy of Sciences.

The **National Academy of Engineering** was established in 1964, under the charter of the National Academy of Sciences, as a parallel organization of outstanding engineers. It is autonomous in its administration and in the selection of its members, sharing with the National Academy of Sciences the responsibility for advising the federal government. The National Academy of Engineering also sponsors engineering programs aimed at meeting national needs, encourages education and research, and recognizes the superior achievements of engineers. Dr. Charles M. Vest is president of the National Academy of Engineering.

The **Institute of Medicine** was established in 1970 by the National Academy of Sciences to secure the services of eminent members of appropriate professions in the examination of policy matters pertaining to the health of the public. The Institute acts under the responsibility given to the National Academy of Sciences by its congressional charter to be an adviser to the federal government and, upon its own initiative, to identify issues of medical care, research, and education. Dr. Harvey V. Fineberg is president of the Institute of Medicine.

The **National Research Council** was organized by the National Academy of Sciences in 1916 to associate the broad community of science and technology with the Academy's purposes of furthering knowledge and advising the federal government. Functioning in accordance with general policies determined by the Academy, the Council has become the principal operating agency of both the National Academy of Sciences and the National Academy of Engineering in providing services to the government, the public, and the scientific and engineering communities. The Council is administered jointly by both Academies and the Institute of Medicine. Dr. Ralph J. Cicerone and Dr. Charles M. Vest are chair and vice chair, respectively, of the National Research Council.

www.national-academies.org

v

OTHER REPORTS OF THE
BOARD ON ENVIRONMENTAL STUDIES AND TOXICOLOGY

Carcinogens and Anticarcinogens in the Human Diet (1996)
Upstream: Salmon and Society in the Pacific Northwest (1996)
Science and the Endangered Species Act (1995)
Wetlands: Characteristics and Boundaries (1995)
Biologic Markers (five volumes, 1989-1995)
Science and Judgment in Risk Assessment (1994)
Pesticides in the Diets of Infants and Children (1993)
Dolphins and the Tuna Industry (1992)
Science and the National Parks (1992)
Human Exposure Assessment for Airborne Pollutants (1991)
Rethinking the Ozone Problem in Urban and Regional Air Pollution (1991)
Decline of the Sea Turtles (1990)

*Copies of these reports may be ordered from the National Academies Press
(800) 624-6242 or (202) 334-3313
www.nap.edu*

Preface

Risk assessments are often focused on a single chemical. People, however, are exposed to mixtures of chemicals over their lifetime, and many argue that a better way to estimate risk is to assess exposure to mixtures, particularly for mixtures of chemicals that have similar mechanisms of toxicity or that produce similar effects. Because phthalates make up a chemical class that produce similar effects and have similar chemical structures, the U.S. Environmental Protection Agency (EPA) asked the National Research Council (NRC) to evaluate their health risks and determine whether a cumulative risk assessment would be appropriate and, if so, suggest an approach to such an assessment.

In this report, the Committee on the Health Risks of Phthalates reviews risk-assessment practices and describes their strengths and weaknesses. The committee reviews the toxicity of and exposure to phthalates, considers the value of conducting a cumulative risk assessment of this chemical class, and provides recommendations for conducting the assessment. Data gaps and research needs are also identified, and the applicability of the committee's recommendations to other chemical classes is discussed.

This report has been reviewed in draft form by persons chosen for their diverse perspectives and technical expertise in accordance with procedures approved by the NRC's Report Review Committee. The purposes of this independent review are to provide candid and critical comments that will assist the institution in making its published report as sound as possible and to ensure that the report meets institutional standards of objectivity, evidence, and responsiveness to the study charge. The review comments and draft manuscript remain confidential to protect the integrity of the deliberative process. We thank the following for their review of this report: Melvin E. Andersen, The Hamner Institutes for Health Sciences; Kenny S. Crump, ENVIRON; Alan R. Boobis, Imperial College London; Ronald Breslow, Columbia University; Patricia A. Buffler, University of California, Berkeley; George P. Daston, Proctor & Gamble Company; John M. DeSesso, Noblis; Holger Koch, Institut der Ruhr-Universität Bochum; William S. Knowles, Monsanto Company (retired); Rochelle Tyl, RTI International; John Wakefield, University of Washington; Paige Williams, Harvard School of Public Health; Lauren A. Zeise, California Environmental Protection Agency.

Although the reviewers listed above have provided many constructive comments and suggestions, they were not asked to endorse the conclusions or recommendations, nor did they see the final draft of the report before its release. The review of the report was overseen by the review coordinator, Thomas A. Louis, Johns Hopkins Bloomberg School of Public Health, and the review monitor, Donald R. Mattison, National Institutes of Health. Appointed by the NRC, they were responsible for making certain that an independent examination of the report was carried out in accordance with institutional procedures and that all review comments were carefully considered. Responsibility for the final content of the report rests entirely with the committee and the institution.

The committee gratefully acknowledges the following for making presentations to the committee: Antonia Calafat, Centers for Disease Control and Prevention; Raymond David, BASF; James Donald, California Environmental Protection Agency; Earl Gray, EPA; Jane Houlihan, Environmental Working Group; Leo Posthuma, RIVM (National Institute of Public Health and the Environment), the Netherlands; Peter Preuss, EPA; Jennifer Sass, Natural Resources Defense Council; Richard Sharpe, Medical Research Council, United Kingdom; Michael Shelby, National Toxicology Program; Jamie Strong, EPA; Shanna Swan, University of Rochester School of Medicine and Dentistry; Linda Teuschler, EPA; and Nigel Walker, National Institute of Environmental Health Sciences.

The committee especially thanks Rebecca Clewell, of the Hamner Institutes for Health Sciences, who provided information on the toxicokinetics of dialkylphthalates that aided the committee in its development of the exposure-assessment chapter, and Earl Gray, of EPA, who provided individual animal data for several toxicity studies that aided the committee in its evaluation of the cumulative risk posed by phthalates.

The committee is also grateful for the assistance of the NRC staff in preparing this report. Staff members who contributed to the effort are Ellen Mantus, project director; James Reisa, director of the Board on Environmental Studies and Toxicology; Norman Grossblatt, senior editor; Mirsada Karalic-Loncarevic, manager, Technical Information Center; Heidi Murray-Smith, research associate; John Brown, program associate; and Panola Golson, senior program assistant.

I would especially like to thank all the members of the committee for their efforts throughout the development of this report.

Deborah Cory-Slechta, *Chair*
Committee on the Health Risks of Phthalates

Contents

BOXES, FIGURES AND TABLES

BOXES

FIGURES

TABLES

Abbreviations

AGD	anogenital distance
AhR	aryl hydrocarbon receptor
AR	androgen receptor
ATSDR	Agency for Toxic Substances and Disease Registry
B[a]P	benzo[a]pyrene
BBP	butyl benzyl phthalate
BMD	benchmark dose
BMDL	lower confidence limit of BMD
BMR	benchmark response
CDC	Centers for Disease Control and Prevention
CERCLA	Comprehensive Environmental Response, Compensation, and Liability Act
CERHR	Center for the Evaluation of Risks to Human Reproduction
CHO	Chinese hamster ovary
CRPF	cumulative relative potency factor
CSF	cancer slope factor
CSL	cranial suspensory ligament
CT	central tendency
DA	dose addition
DBP	di-*n*-butyl phthalate
DCHP	dicyclohexyl phthalate
DDT	dichloro-diphenyl-trichloroethane
DEHP	di(2-ethylhexyl) phthalate
DEP	diethyl phthalate
DHT	dihydrotestosterone
DIBP	diisobutyl phthalate
DIDP	diisodecyl phthalate
DINP	diisononyl phthalate
DMP	dimethyl phthalate
DMT	dimethyl terephthalate or dimethyl-*p*-phthalate
DOP	di-*n*-octyl phthalate
DPHP	di(2-propylheptyl) phthalate
DPP	dipentyl phthalate
ECAO	Environmental Criteria and Assessment Office
ED_x	effective dose at x response level

EPA	U.S. Environmental Protection Agency
EU	European Union
FSH	follicle-stimulating hormone
GD	gestation day
Gub	gubernaculum
HI	hazard index
HQ	hazard quotient
IA	independent action
insl3	insulin-like factor 3
IQ	intelligence quotient
IQR	interquartile range
IRIS	Integrated Risk Information System
LABC	levator ani/bulbocavernosus muscles
LC	Leydig cell
LOAEL	lowest observed-adverse-effect level
LOD	limit of detection
LOEL	lowest observed-effect level
MADL	maximum allowable dose level
MBP	monobutyl phthalate
MBZP	monobenzyl phthalate
MCHP	monocyclohexyl phthalate
MCINP	mono(carboxyisononyl) phthalate
MCIOP	mono(carboxyisooctyl) phthalate
MCPHP	mono(carboxypropylheptyl) phthalate
MCPP	mono-3-carboxypropyl phthalate
MECPP	mono(2-ethyl-5-carboxypentyl) phthalate
MEHHP	mono(2-ethyl-5-hydroxyhexyl) phthalate
MEHP	mono(2-ethylhexyl) phthalate
MEOHP	mono(2-ethyl-5-oxohexyl) phthalate
MEP	monoethyl phthalate
MHIDP	mono(hydroxyisodecyl) phthalate
MHINP	mono(hydroxyisononyl) phthalate
MHPHP	mono(hydroxypropylheptyl) phthalate
MIBP	monoisobutyl phthalate
MIDP	monoisodecyl phthalate
MINP	monoisononyl phthalate
MIS	Mullerian inhibiting substance
MMP	monomethyl phthalate
MOIDP	mono(oxoisodecyl) phthalate
MOINP	mono(oxoisononyl) phthalate
MOP	mono-*n*-octyl phthalate
MOPHP	mono(oxopropylheptyl) phthalate
MPHP	monopropylheptyl phthalate
MRL	minimal risk level
NATA	National Air Toxics Assessment

NHANES	National Health and Nutrition Examination Survey
NOAEL	no-observed-adverse-effect level
NOEL	no-observed-effect level
NR	nipple retention
NRC	National Research Council
NTP	National Toxicology Program
p,p'-DDE	*p,p'*-dichlorodiphenyl dichloroethylene
PAH	polycyclic aromatic hydrocarbon
PBDE	polybrominated diphenyl ethers
PBPK	physiologically based pharmacokinetic
PCB	polychlorinated biphenyls
PCDD	polychlorinated dibenzo-*p*-dioxins
PCDF	polychlorinated dibenzo-*p*-furans
POD	point of departure
PPARα	peroxisome-proliferator-activated receptor-α
PPRTV	provisional peer reviewed toxicity value
RAGS	Risk Assessment Guidance for Superfund
RfC	reference concentration
RfD	reference dose
RME	reasonable maximum exposure
S.V.	seminal vesicles
STSC	Superfund Health Risk Technical Support Center
TCDD	tetrachlorodibenzo-*p*-dioxin
TCP/TAL	Contract Laboratory Program Target Compound and Target Analyte List
TDS	testicular dysgenesis syndrome
TEF	toxicity equivalence factor
TEQ	toxic equivalence
UR	unit risk

PHTHALATES
AND CUMULATIVE
RISK ASSESSMENT

The Tasks Ahead

Summary

People are exposed to a great variety of chemicals throughout their daily lives in the foods they eat, in the air they breathe, and in the water they drink. Some exposures, such as to natural components of foods, are clearly intentional, and others are inadvertent. Over the last few decades, the U.S. Environmental Protection Agency (EPA) has been developing guidance to evaluate the cumulative risk posed by multiple chemical exposures and other stressors that can modify the effects of specific chemical exposures. Recent guidance has tended to focus on chemicals that are structurally related, such as organophosphate pesticides, on the assumption that such chemicals have a common mechanism of action.

Phthalate esters constitute a chemical class about which concern has emerged. Phthalates are used in a wide variety of consumer products, including cosmetics, personal-care products, pharmaceuticals, medical devices, children's toys, food packaging, and cleaning and building materials. Recent studies show widespread human exposure to multiple phthalates and indicate that effects on the development of the reproductive system of laboratory animals occur at much lower doses than were predicted in earlier studies. The European Union and the United States have passed legislation that restricts the concentrations of several phthalates in children's toys, and the European Union has banned several phthalates from cosmetics. In this context, EPA asked the National Research Council to review independently the health effects of phthalates, determine whether cumulative risk assessment of this chemical class should be conducted, and, if so, indicate approaches that could be used for the assessment. The applicability of such approaches to other chemical classes and to cumulative risk assessment generally was also to be considered. In response to EPA's request, the National Research Council convened the Committee on the Health Risks of Phthalates, which prepared this report.

To address its task, the committee reviewed scientific literature on phthalates and the effects of chemical mixtures, reviewed guidance and other documents on cumulative risk assessment, and heard presentations by experts in the fields of phthalate toxicity and cumulative risk. The committee found that the definition of cumulative risk assessment has evolved over the years but agreed with recent publications that define cumulative risk broadly to mean the risk posed by multiple chemicals and other stressors that cause varied health effects and to which people are exposed by multiple pathways and exposure routes and for varied durations.

This report is not a comprehensive toxicologic profile or risk assessment of any particular phthalate or of the chemical class as a whole. Rather, it answers two questions: Should cumulative risk assessment of phthalates be conducted? If so, how should the assessment be conducted? The committee considered primarily the most sensitive health outcomes resulting from exposure to phthalates (effects on the development of the male reproductive system) as an illustrative example for cumulative risk assessment. The committee's suggestions should not be interpreted to imply that other health effects are not important or that nonchemical stressors should be ignored.

MODE OF ACTION, MECHANISM OF ACTION, AND COMMON ADVERSE OUTCOMES

Mode of action and *mechanism of action* are terms that are commonly used in risk assessment and often used interchangeably. Both refer to the biologic pathway to some final health outcome; the difference between the terms is the level of detail used to describe the pathway. Typically, *mechanism of action* is used to describe the pathway at the molecular level, and *mode of action* is used to describe the key events along the pathway. Although the committee recognizes the distinction and does not want to contribute to greater confusion concerning the use of the terms, *mechanism of action* is used in this report to describe the biologic pathway.

In recent years, the focus in cumulative risk assessment has been on chemicals that have common mechanisms of action. As described below and in greater detail in this report, the committee finds that the focus in cumulative risk assessment should be on the health outcomes and not on the pathways that lead to them, whether defined as mechanisms of action or as modes of action. Multiple pathways can lead to a common outcome, and a focus on only a specific pathway can lead to too narrow an approach in conducting a cumulative risk assessment. Accordingly, the chemicals that should be considered for cumulative risk assessment should be ones that cause the same health outcomes or the same types of health outcomes, such as a specific set of effects on male reproductive development, not ones that cause the health outcomes only by a specific pathway. The committee refers to the health outcomes of interest as *common adverse outcomes*.

WHY A CUMULATIVE RISK ASSESSMENT?

Answering two basic questions helps to determine whether a cumulative risk assessment of phthalates is warranted. First, are there exposures to multiple phthalates? Second, do the exposures contribute to common adverse outcomes? There is clearly potential for exposures because phthalates occur in a wide variety of consumer products, including toys, cosmetics, pharmaceuticals, and building and construction materials. Furthermore, the National Health and Nutrition Examination Survey (NHANES) conducted by the Centers for Disease Control and Prevention has documented simultaneous exposure to multiple phthalates in the general population, including children and adults. Other studies support those findings. An important finding of the surveys is that concentrations of phthalate metabolites in urine are generally higher in children than adults; the differences may result from differences in exposure or from possible differences in metabolism between children and adults. The metabolic differences are important because they may alter the risk posed by exposure; that is, they may make one person more or less susceptible than another to the effects of phthalates. Other studies have shown that phthalates cross the placenta, and multiple phthalates have been measured in animal and human amniotic fluid. On the basis of the exposure surveys and studies, the first question—whether there is exposure to multiple phthalates—has been answered affirmatively. Not only concurrent exposure, but concurrent exposure at all life stages, has been demonstrated.

The second question concerns whether exposures to multiple phthalates contribute to common adverse outcomes. Few human data on the health effects of phthalate exposure are available. Most data are from laboratory studies of rats, which have been shown to be the most phthalate-sensitive of the species tested. Early studies indicated that hepatic cancer and teratogenic effects could be induced if high doses were administered long enough or during a specific time. However, the protocol of the early teratology studies required dosing pregnant animals from gestation day 6 to 15 (the major period of organogenesis). In the late 1990s, it became evident that chemicals could affect sexual differentiation, which occurs during gestation days 12-21 in rats. Thus, the early protocol did not expose animals throughout the critical developmental window. The time when the animals were evaluated also posed a problem. The standard teratology protocol requires that fetuses be examined just before term; however, the malformations characteristic of phthalate exposure would be difficult or impossible to diagnose without a detailed histopathologic examination, which is not required by current guidelines. If the protocol is modified to include exposure during the critical window and the animals are examined postnatally, a variety of effects on the development of the reproductive system can be observed in males at much lower doses than previously observed after exposure to various phthalates. That group of effects observed in male animals is known as the phthalate syndrome and includes infertility, decreased sperm count, crypt-orchidism (undescended testes), hypospadias (malformation of the penis in which the urethra does not open at the tip of the organ), and other reproductive tract malformations. Those effects are characteristic more generally of distur-bance of androgen[1] action. Furthermore, the phthalate syndrome has many simi-larities to the hypothesized testicular dysgenesis syndrome in humans, although there are no human data that directly link the hypothesized syndrome with phthalate exposure.

Figure S-1 shows the relationship between the various syndromes and il-lustrates the range of common effects on the development of the male reproduc-tive system. The committee concludes that the second question—about common adverse outcomes of phthalates—has been answered affirmatively. However, the committee emphasizes that not all phthalates are equivalent in the severity of their effects. The phthalates that are most potent in causing effects on the devel-opment of the male reproductive system are generally those with ester chains of four to six carbon atoms; phthalates with shorter or longer chains typically ex-hibit less severe or no effects. Furthermore, the age of the animals at the time of

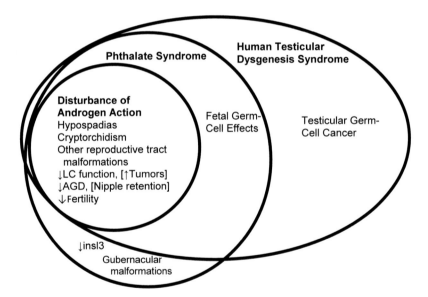

FIGURE S-1 Relationship of phthalate syndrome in rats to effects associated with agents that perturb androgen action and produce androgen insufficiency and to the hypothesized testicular dysgenesis syndrome in humans. Outcomes in brackets are restricted to findings in experimental animals. AGD, anogenital distance; insl3, insulin-like factor 3; LC, Ley-dig cell; ↑, increase; and ↓, decrease.

[1]*Androgen* is a generic term for male sex hormone. The primary androgen is testoster-one.

exposure is critical with respect to the severity of the effects; the fetus is the most sensitive life stage.

Studies indicate that some phthalates reduce testosterone concentrations; this androgen insufficiency causes the variety of effects observed if it occurs at times that are critical for male reproductive development. That point is important in considering cumulative risk assessment because a number of other agents (often referred to as antiandrogens) can produce similar effects through perturbations in androgen concentrations or in androgen-receptor signaling. In reproductive tissues that require androgen for normal development, it is unlikely that one can differentiate between a decreased concentration of androgen and antagonism of androgen-receptor signaling; the responses would be similar. Thus, any agent that can produce androgen insufficiency or block androgen-receptor signaling in the developing male fetus would have effects that are included in the array of malformations known to be caused by phthalates.

On the basis of the findings summarized above, the committee recommends that a cumulative risk assessment be conducted for phthalates and that the assessment include other antiandrogens, as described further in the next section.

CONSIDERATIONS FOR CONDUCTING CUMULATIVE RISK ASSESSMENT

One approach to cumulative risk assessment of a mixture is to consider the mixture as a single agent and develop toxicity data on the mixture. That approach has been used for some industrial products, such as commercial mixtures of polychlorinated biphenyls, and industrial waste streams, such as coke-oven emissions. However, such an approach assumes that the composition of the mixture does not change and that the components always occur together. Because the components and concentrations of phthalate mixtures are likely to vary, the whole-mixture approach is not appropriate for phthalates.

Another approach is to explain the effects of a mixture in terms of the individual components (that is, a component-based approach). When chemicals in a mixture act together to produce an effect and do not enhance or diminish each other's actions, the outcome of exposure to the mixture is considered additive. Two distinct concepts—dose addition and independent action[2]—have been used as models to describe and estimate ideal additive mixture effects, although other approaches have been introduced, and the literature can be confusing and may often appear contradictory. Dose addition arises if the "dilution" principle applies, so that one chemical can be replaced with a fraction of an equally effective concentration of another chemical without changing the overall combined effect. Independent action is based on the idea of, and may arise from, statistically independent action of each component. Mixtures may demonstrate effects larger than expected (synergism) or smaller than expected (antagonism), although the

---

[2]Independent action is also referred to as response addition.

determination of synergism or antagonism may depend on the model chosen for comparison.

There are marked differences between the chemical-by-chemical approach to risk assessment and evaluations that take mixture effects into account. Where single-chemical risk assessments might yield the verdict "absence of risk," dose addition might yield the opposite conclusion. Specifically, there is an expectation with dose addition that every component at any dose contributes, in proportion to its prevalence, to the overall mixture toxicity. Whether the individual doses of mixture components are effective on their own does not matter. For example, let a dose of 4×10^{-2} arbitrary dose units produce an effect of measurable magnitude (see Figure S-2). The same effect will be obtained when the chemical is administered in 10 simultaneous portions of 4×10^{-3} dose units, even though the response to each one of those dose fractions is not measurable. If dose addition applies, the same holds when 10 portions of 10 chemicals with identical response curves are used. Thus, combined effects should also result from chemicals at doses associated with no measurable effect or "zero" effect, provided that sufficiently large numbers of components sum to a suitably high effect dose. The situation described here for dose addition may not be the case with independent action because responses are viewed "independently" of each other, and summing "zero" effects of the individual components would lead to a

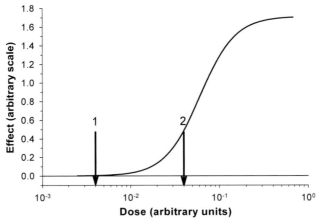

FIGURE S-2 Illustration of a hypothetical mixture experiment with chemicals that all exhibit the same dose-response curve. At the low dose to the left (arrow 1, 4×10^{-3} dose units), the effect is hardly observable. A combination of 10 agents at that dose (arrow 2, total dose, 4×10^{-2} dose units) produces a significant combined effect consistent with expectations based on dose addition.

prediction of a "zero" mixture effect. However, that proposition forces clear distinctions between "zero" effects and small effects that are beyond the resolving power of experimental studies. Particularly in the case of mixtures of large numbers of components, small, albeit statistically insignificant responses may sum to considerable mixture effects, even when independent action applies.

Various EPA programs and offices have developed cumulative-risk-assessment definitions and approaches that are specific to their regulatory or statutory needs, although early guidance focused on dose-addition methods as a default, at least for chemicals that affect a given organ system. Recent EPA guidance has asserted that if dose-addition methods are to be used, the chemicals for consideration should exhibit the same mechanism of action. However, it can be difficult to define criteria for determining similar mechanisms of action. Some might say that chemicals that produce similar responses have the same mechanism of action, and others might require that data show that chemicals act through identical molecular pathways and thus produce exactly the same intermediates at each step in the pathway. The latter requirement would result in consideration of few chemicals for any cumulative risk assessment. EPA also stipulates in recent guidance documents that dose-response curves of the chemicals should be parallel if dose-addition methods are to be used.

The committee concluded that EPA's more recent stipulations on when dose-addition methods should be used are too restrictive. Phthalates may not all act by the same mechanisms, and they do not have parallel dose-response curves. However, those facts do not negate the appropriateness of using general dose-addition methods in a cumulative risk assessment. The committee emphasizes that parallel dose-response curves are not required for dose-addition methods generally, although they may be required for some specific applications, such as some relative-potency approaches.

The stipulations that EPA has placed on using dose-addition methods raise a greater issue. The stipulations have affected how EPA evaluates chemicals for cumulative risk assessment, for example, grouping structurally related chemicals on the assumption that they act by the same mechanisms. For cumulative risk assessment, the committee strongly recommends that EPA group chemicals that cause common adverse outcomes and not focus exclusively on structural similarity or on similar mechanisms of action. Accordingly, phthalates *and other agents* that cause androgen insufficiency or block androgen-receptor signaling, and are thus capable of inducing effects that characterize components of the phthalate syndrome, should be considered in a cumulative risk assessment. A focus solely on phthalates to the exclusion of other antiandrogens would be artificial and could seriously underestimate cumulative risk.

The question then becomes whether dose addition, independent action, or some other method is the most appropriate for estimating risk associated with phthalates and other antiandrogens. The committee concludes that the answer should be based on empirical data that directly test any proposed method. Mixture studies in laboratory animals have been conducted with phthalates, with other antiandrogens, and with phthalates *and* other antiandrogens; the results all indicate that the mixture effects in each case are predicted well with dose-addition methods. Although a variety of mechanisms clearly are involved, dose addition proved adequately predictive when the committee evaluated the available data. More important, when the model predictions differed significantly, no case could be found in which independent action predicted mixture effects better than dose addition. Thus, the evidence supports the use of dose addition as an approximation in estimating cumulative risk posed by phthalates and other antiandrogens. The use of a dose-addition model is also supported by data that show cumulative effects at doses at which individual mixture components did not induce observable effects.

There are several approaches for conducting cumulative risk assessment with the dose-addition approach. This report outlines a few possible options, ranging from the relatively straightforward, focusing on one particular outcome, to the more complex, involving the development of a composite score for a variety of outcomes. Each option will have advantages and disadvantages, and EPA should evaluate each option and determine which is most appropriate. The committee emphasizes that the conceptual approach taken for phthalates should be applicable to other agents.

FUTURE DIRECTIONS

The current practice of restricting cumulative risk assessment to structurally or mechanistically related chemicals ignores the important fact that different chemical exposures may result in the same common adverse outcomes. Focusing primarily on physiologic consequences rather than structural or mechanistic similarity is a critical and achievable next step in cumulative risk assessment and is more directly relevant to relating chemical exposures to human diseases and disorders. Accordingly, the cumulative risk assessment of phthalates should consider any chemical that leads to disturbance of androgen action and is thus capable of inducing any of the effects on the development of the male reproductive system that are characteristic of phthalate exposure (see Figure S-3). Which chemicals to include in the cumulative risk assessment will depend on whether there is a potential for exposure in which the chemicals would exhibit common adverse outcomes. The committee emphasizes that its recommendation to focus on common adverse outcomes in cumulative risk assessment does not mean that information on mechanism of action is not desirable. That information is useful for defining critical pathways and system-level physiology, for determining the relevance of effects observed in animals to humans, and for reducing uncertainty in determining risk.

On the basis of its review, the committee concludes that sufficient data are available to proceed with the cumulative risk assessment of phthalates and other antiandrogens. However, addressing current data gaps would lead to greater refinement of a cumulative risk assessment and reduce uncertainty associated

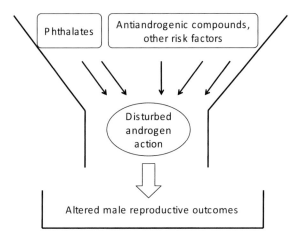

FIGURE S-3 Multiple exposures leading to common adverse outcomes.

with any risk estimates. Because issues surrounding fetal exposure are particularly important in phthalate risk assessment, research to determine prenatal exposure to phthalates at multiple relevant times during pregnancy is critical. It is especially important to determine whether metabolite concentrations in the fetal compartment vary during pregnancy; if they do, it would indicate possible metabolic differences at different gestational ages. More generally, the full spectrum of phthalate metabolites needs to be characterized, the most appropriate metabolites to use as biomarkers of human exposure need to be determined, and the most important sources of phthalate exposure in the general population need to be identified. Because differences in susceptibility clearly depend on age, species, and exposure route, research to understand why the differences occur is important. Finally, research is needed to investigate possible deviations from the dose-addition concept—that is, identification of cases of synergism or antagonism relative to dose addition.

The committee recognizes that its recommendation to move beyond the constraints of structural or mechanistic similarity for cumulative risk assessment may appear challenging. One might ask, "With so many chemicals, where do we begin?" However, the committee concludes that it is plausible and warranted to extend cumulative risk assessment to include chemicals associated with common adverse outcomes as exemplified in this report by inclusion of other antiandrogenic chemicals with phthalates. To cite another example, EPA could evaluate combined exposures to lead, methylmercury, and polychlorinated biphenyls because all contribute to cumulative risk of cognitive deficits consistent with IQ reduction in children, although the deficits are produced by different mechanisms of action. Cumulative risk assessment based on common adverse outcomes is a feasible and physiologically relevant approach to the evaluation of the multiplicity of human exposures and directly reflects EPA's mission to protect human health. Such a shift in approach would entail substantial efforts by EPA, such as those required to define and set priorities among the most important adverse health outcomes. However, a focus on common adverse outcomes actually facilitates the process by defining the groups of agents that should be included for a given outcome.

1

Introduction

Humans are exposed to a variety of chemicals at any one time, and the exposures change over time. Recognition of the dynamic and varied nature of chemical exposures has prompted a growing emphasis on assessing risks in a cumulative manner. In 1986, the U.S. Environmental Protection Agency (EPA) published *Guidelines for the Health Risk Assessment of Chemical Mixtures*, and over the years, the progression toward a cumulative risk paradigm has prompted the publication of several frameworks and guidance documents for conducting cumulative risk assessment (ILSI 1999; EPA 1997, 2000, 2002, 2003, 2006, 2007). Some methods have focused on structurally related chemicals on the assumption that they act through a common mechanism of action. Examples include the development of toxic equivalency factors for dioxins (EPA 1987, 1989; Van den Berg et al. 2006) and polychlorinated biphenyls (Van den Berg et al. 2006) and the development of relative potency factors for polycyclic aromatic hydrocarbons (EPA 1993) and cholinesterase-inhibiting organophosphate pesticides (EPA 2002).

Phthalates are a group of chemicals with similar chemical structure that have been associated with effects on the development of the reproductive system of male laboratory animals. Few epidemiologic studies of phthalates and developmental effects on the male reproductive system are available; however, studies show widespread human exposures to phthalates. Those and other factors prompted EPA to ask that the National Research Council (NRC) assess the appropriateness of conducting a cumulative risk assessment of this chemical class and provide guidance for such an assessment as related not only to phthalates but to cumulative risk assessment generally. This report provides the conclusions and recommendations of the Committee on the Health Risks of Phthalates established by the NRC in response to EPA's request.

PHTHALATES

Phthalates are diesters of benzenedicarboxylic acid. The committee restricted its assessment to the most biologically active phthalates, diesters of 1,2-

benzenedicarboxylic acid, or *o*-phthalates, which have the general chemical structure shown in Figure 1-1. Throughout this report, the term *phthalates* refers to the *o*-phthalates unless otherwise indicated.

The ester side chains can vary in length and structure. For example, they can be identical as in the case of di-*n*-butyl phthalate (R and R' are both $-CH_2 CH_2CH_2CH_3$), or they can differ as in the case of butyl benzyl phthalate (R is $-CH_2CH_2CH_2CH_3$, and R' is $-CH_2C_6H_5$). The structural differences in the ester side chains give the phthalates their individual chemical and physical properties and alter their biologic activity. Table 1-1 lists common phthalates and selected metabolites. The abbreviations provided in Table 1-1 are used throughout this report.

Phthalates are used to impart flexibility to plastics and for their solvent properties. They are used in a wide variety of consumer products, including cosmetics, personal-care products, pharmaceuticals, medical devices, children's toys, food packaging, and cleaning and building materials (Schettler 2006). The widespread use of phthalates has raised concerns regarding potential human exposure. As part of the 1999-2000 National Health and Nutrition Examination Survey (NHANES), the Centers for Disease Control and Prevention (CDC) measured several phthalate monoesters (metabolites of the diesters) in urine (Silva et al. 2004). Later surveys have provided additional data on phthalate exposure (CDC 2007a,b). Those and other surveys indicate widespread human exposure to various phthalates (Hauser and Calafat 2005).

Phthalate exposures can produce a variety of effects in laboratory animals; however, their adverse effects on the development of the reproductive system of male animals have led to particular concern. The effects of fetal exposure of male laboratory animals include infertility, decreased sperm count, crypt-orchidism (undescended testes), hypospadias (malformation of the penis in which the urethra does not open at the tip of the organ), and other reproductive tract malformations and are similar to those that characterize the hypothesized testicular dysgenesis syndrome in humans (Skakkebæk et al. 2001). Currently, epidemiologic evidence of adverse human health effects of phthalate exposure is inadequate or limited (Hauser and Calafat 2005). Recently, the European Union

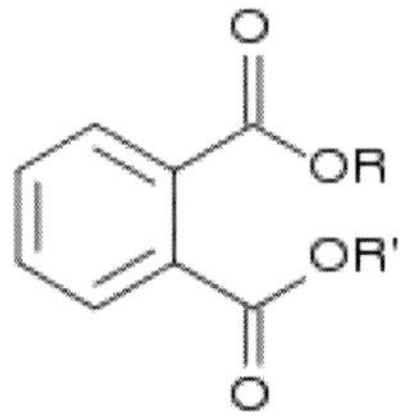

FIGURE 1-1 General chemical structure of an *o*-phthalate.

TABLE 1-1 Phthalate Parent Compounds and Selected Metabolites

Phthalate		CAS Registry Number	Molecular Weight	Selected Metabolites	
DMP	dimethyl phthalate	131-11-3	194	MMP	monomethyl phthalate
DEP	diethyl phthalate	84-66-2	222	MEP	monoethyl phthalate
DBP	di-*n*-butyl phthalate	84-74-2	278	MBP	monobutyl phthalate
DIBP	diisobutyl phthalate	84-69-5	278	MIBP	monoisobutyl phthalate
BBP	butyl benzyl phthalate	85-68-7	312	MBZP	monobenzyl phthalate
DCHP	dicyclohexyl phthalate	84-61-7	330	MCHP	monocyclohexyl phthalate
DEHP	di(2-ethylhexyl) phthalate	117-81-7	390	MECPP	mono(2-ethyl-5-carboxypentyl) phthalate
				MEOHP	mono(2-ethyl-5-oxohexyl) phthalate
				MEHHP	mono(2-ethyl-5-hydroxyhexyl) phthalate
				MEHP	mono(2-ethylhexyl) phthalate
DOP	di-*n*-octyl phthalate	117-84-0	390	MCPP	mono-3-carboxypropyl phthalate
				MOP	mono-*n*-octyl phthalate

(Continued)

TABLE 1-1 Continued

Phthalate		CAS Registry Number	Molecular Weight	Selected Metabolites	
DINP	diisononyl phthalate	28553-12-0	419	MCIOP	mono(carboxyisooctyl) phthalate
				MHINP	mono(hydroxyisononyl) phthalate
				MOINP	mono(oxoisononyl) phthalate
				MINP	monoisononyl phthalate
DIDP	diisodecyl phthalate	26761-40-0	447	MCINP	mono(carboxyisononyl) phthalate
				MHIDP	mono(hydroxyisodecyl) phthalate
				MOIDP	mono(oxoisodecyl) phthalate
				MIDP	monoisodecyl phthalate
DPHP	di(2-propylheptyl) phthalate	53306-54-0	447	MCPHP	mono(carboxypropylheptyl) phthalate
				MHPHP	mono(hydroxypropylheptyl) phthalate
				MOPHP	mono(oxopropylheptyl) phthalate
				MPHP	monopropylheptyl phthalate

(EU 2005a) and the United States[1] have passed legislation that restricts the concentration of selected phthalates in children's toys, and the European Union has banned several phthalates from cosmetics (EU 2004, 2005b).

THE COMMITTEE'S TASK AND APPROACH

The widespread human exposure to phthalates coupled with the ability of this chemical class to induce male reproductive toxicity in laboratory animals prompted EPA's request to the NRC to conduct an independent scientific evaluation of phthalates in the context of cumulative risk assessment. Specifically, the committee was asked to review critical scientific data and address questions related to the human relevance of experimental data, modes of action, exposure information, dose-response relationships, and the potential for cumulative effects. The committee was further asked to consider the strengths and weaknesses of cumulative-assessment approaches, to provide recommendations to EPA on conducting a cumulative risk assessment of phthalate chemicals, and to identify additional research needs. Finally, the committee was asked to consider the applicability of its recommendations to cumulative risk assessment of other chemical classes. See Appendix A for a verbatim statement of task. Given the statement of task, the committee members were selected for their expertise in biostatistics, epidemiology, exposure assessment, toxicology, pediatrics, risk assessment, cumulative risk assessment, and risk management. See Appendix B for biographic information on the committee.

To accomplish its task, the committee held five meetings from December 2007 to June 2008. In public sessions during the first two meetings, the committee heard presentations from the sponsor and invited speakers from government agencies, academe, industry, and environmental groups. The committee reviewed numerous scientific publications on cumulative risk assessment, phthalate exposure, and phthalate toxicity. The committee first focused on the central question of whether a cumulative risk assessment is appropriate for the phthalate esters. Given the committee's agreement that a cumulative risk assessment was warranted, it focused on approaches to such an assessment. Particular weight was given to approaches that would help the process to evolve and would be applicable to the real-world context in which humans are exposed to a variety of structurally and nonstructurally related chemicals. Accordingly, this report is not a comprehensive toxicologic profile, nor is it a cumulative risk assessment, of phthalates. Furthermore, although the committee clearly recognized that cumulative risk assessment must encompass the assessment of multiple agents and other stressors to which people are exposed by multiple pathways and routes and for varied durations and that cause varied health effects, it restricted its examination to the most sensitive outcomes (that is, effects on the development of the male reproductive system) exhibited in laboratory animals as a result of phthal-

---

[1]Consumer Product Safety Improvement Act of 2008, Title II §108 (a)(b) (H.R. 4040).

ate exposure. As a final consideration, the committee evaluated the applicability of the proposed approaches to other chemical classes and more broadly to chemicals that produce common adverse outcomes.

ORGANIZATION OF THE REPORT

The committee's report is organized into six chapters and four appendixes. Chapter 2 summarizes sources and routes of phthalate exposure, reviews available exposure data, and discusses phthalate metabolism. Chapter 3 reviews toxicity, particularly developmental toxicity in the male reproductive system, that results from phthalate exposure. Chapter 4 provides a synopsis of current risk-assessment practices and identifies their strengths and weaknesses. Chapter 5 addresses whether a cumulative risk assessment is appropriate for phthalates, recommends approaches for such an assessment, and discusses the applicability of the approaches to other chemicals. Chapter 6 identifies needed data and research that could help to refine a cumulative risk assessment of phthalates and reduce the associated uncertainty. Appendix A is the verbatim statement of task, Appendix B provides biographic information on the committee, Appendix C provides the committee's reanalysis of some phthalate-mixture data, and Appendix D is a case study that illustrates one risk-assessment approach suggested by the committee.

REFERENCES

CDC (Centers for Disease Control and Prevention). 2007a. National Health and Nutrition Examination Survey Data: 2001-2002. U.S. Department of Health and Human Services, Centers for Disease Control and Prevention, National Center for Health Statistics, Hyattsville, MD [online]. Available: http://www.cdc.gov/nchs/about/major/nhanes/nhanes01-02.htm [accessed June 10, 2008].

CDC (Centers for Disease Control and Prevention). 2007b. National Health and Nutrition Examination Survey Data: 2003-2004. U.S. Department of Health and Human Services, Centers for Disease Control and Prevention, National Center for Health Statistics, Hyattsville, MD [online]. Available: http://www.cdc.gov/nchs/about/major/nhanes/nhanes2003-2004/nhanes03_04.htm [accessed June 10, 2008].

EPA (U.S. Environmental Protection Agency). 1986. Guidelines for the Health Risk Assessment of Chemical Mixtures. EPA/630/R-98/002. Risk Assessment Forum, U.S. Environmental Protection Agency, Washington, DC. September 1986 [online]. Available: http://www.epa.gov/NCEA/raf/pdfs/chem_mix/chemmix_1986. pdf [accessed Aug. 11, 2008].

EPA (U.S. Environmental Protection Agency). 1987. Interim Procedures for Estimating Risks Associated with Exposures to Mixtures of Chlorinated Dibenzo-*p*-Dioxins and -Dibenzofurans (CDDs and CDFs). EPA/625/3-87/012. Risk Assessment Forum, U.S. Environmental Protection Agency, Washington, DC [online]. Available: http://nepis.epa.gov/Exe/ZyPURL.cgi?Dockey=20007V43.txt [accessed Nov. 12, 2008].

EPA (U.S. Environmental Protection Agency). 1989. Interim Procedures for Estimating Risks Associated with Exposures to Mixtures of Chlorinated Dibenzo-*p*-Dioxins and -Dibenzofurans (CDDs and CDFs) and 1989 Update. EPA/625/3-89/016. Risk Assessment Forum, U.S. Environmental Protection Agency, Washington, DC. March 1989 [online]. Available: http://nepis.epa.gov/Exe/ZyPURL.cgi?Dockey= 300047JJ.txt [accessed Nov. 12, 2008].

EPA (U.S. Environmental Protection Agency). 1993. Provisional Guidance for Quantitative Risk Assessment of Polycyclic Aromatic Hydrocarbons. EPA/600/R-93/089. Office of Research and Development, U.S. Environmental Protection Agency, Washington, DC. July 1993 [online]. Available: http://www.epa.gov/oswer/ riskassessment/pdf/1993_epa_600_r-93_c89.pdf [accessed June 10, 2008].

EPA (U.S. Environmental Protection Agency). 1997. Guidance on Cumulative Risk Assessment. Part I Planning and Scoping, EPA Science Policy Council, July 3, 1997, and Memo from the EPA Administrator, July 3, 1997 [online]. Available: http://www.epa.gov/OSA/spc/pdfs/cumrisk2.pdf and http://www.epa.gov/OSA/ spc/pdfs/cumulrisk.pdf [accessed July 13, 2008].

EPA (U.S. Environmental Protection Agency). 2000. Supplementary Guidance for Conducting Health Risk Assessment of Chemical Mixtures. EPA/630/R-00/002. Risk Assessment Forum, U.S. Environmental Protection Agency, Washington, DC. August 2000 [online]. Available: http://www.epa.gov/NCEA/raf/pdfs/chem_mix/ chem_mix_08_2001.pdf [accessed June 10, 2008].

EPA (U.S. Environmental Protection Agency). 2002. Guidance on Cumulative Risk Assessment of Pesticide Chemicals That Have a Common Mechanism of Toxicity. Office of Pesticide Programs, U.S. Environmental Protection Agency, Washington, DC. January 14, 2002 [online]. Available: http://www.epa.gov/oppfead1/trac/ science/cumulative_guidance.pdf [accessed June 10, 2008].

EPA (U.S. Environmental Protection Agency). 2003. Framework for Cumulative Risk Assessment. EPA/630/P-02/001F. Risk Assessment Forum, U.S. Environmental Protection Agency, Washington, DC. May 2003 [online]. Available: oaspub.epa. gov/eims/eimscomm.getfile?p_download_id=36941 [accessed June 10, 2008].

EPA (U.S. Environmental Protection Agency). 2006. Considerations for Developing Alternative Health Risk Assessment Approaches for Addressing Multiple Chemicals, Exposures and Effects (External Review Draft). EPA/600/R-06/013A. National Center for Environmental Assessment, Office of Research and Development, U.S. Environmental Protection Agency, Cincinnati, OH. March 2006 [online]. Available: http://cfpub.epa.gov/ncea/cfm/recordisplay.cfm?deid=149983 [accessed June 2008].

EPA (U.S. Environmental Protection Agency). 2007. Concepts, Methods, and Data Sources for Cumulative Health Risk Assessment of Multiple Chemicals, Exposures and Effects: A Resource Document. EPA/600/R-06/013F. National Center for Environmental Assessment, Office of Research and Development, U.S. Environmental Protection Agency, Cincinnati, OH, in collaboration with U.S. Department of Energy, Argonne National Laboratory, Environmental Assessment Division, Argonne, IL. August 2007 [online]. Available: http://cfpub.epa.gov/ncea/ cfm/recordisplay.cfm?deid=190187 [accessed Nov. 12, 2008].

EU (European Union). 2004. Commission Directive 2004/93/EC of 21 September 2004 Amending Council Directive 76/768/EEC for the Purpose of Adapting its Annexes II and III to Technical Progress. Official Journal of European Union I.300:13-41. Sept. 25, 2004 [online]. Available: http://ec.europa.eu/enterprise/cosmetics/doc/ 2004_93/en.pdf [accessed Oct. 21, 2008].

EU (European Union). 2005a. Directive 2005/84/EC of the European Parliament and of the Council 14 December 2005 amending for the 22nd time Council Directive 76/769/EEC on the approximation of the laws, regulations and administrative provisions of the Member States relating to restrictions on the marketing and use of certain dangerous substances and preparations (phthalates in toys and childcare articles). Official Journal of the European Union L344:40-43. December 27, 2005 [online]. Available: http://eur-lex.europa.eu/LexUriServ/LexUriServ.do?uri=OJ: L:2005:344:0040:0043:EN:PDF [accessed April 1, 2008].

EU (European Union). 2005b. Commission Directive 2005/80/EC of 21 November 2005 Amending Council Directive 76/768/EEC, Concerning Cosmetic Products, for the Purposes of Adapting Annexes II and III there to Technical Progress. Official Journal of European Union I. 303:32-37. Nov. 22, 2005 [online]. Available: http://ec.europa.eu/enterprise/cosmetics/doc/2005_80/dir_2005_80_en.pdf [accessed Oct. 21, 2008].

Hauser, R., and A.M. Calafat. 2005. Phthalates and human health. Occup. Environ. Med. 62(11):806-818.

ILSI (International Life Sciences Institute). 1999. A Framework for Cumulative Risk Assessment: An ILSI Risk Science Institute Workshop Report, B. Mileson, E. Faustman, S. Olin, P.B. Ryan, S. Ferenc, and T. Burke, eds. ILSI Press, Washington, DC: ILSI Press [online]. Available: http://rsi.ilsi.org/file/rsiframrpt.pdf [accessed June 10, 2008].

Schettler, T. 2006. Human exposure to phthalates via consumer products. Int. J. Androl. 29(1):134-139.

Silva, M.J., D.B. Barr, J.A. Reidy, N.A. Malek,, C.C. Hodge, S.P. Caudill, J.W. Brock, L.L. Needham, and A.M. Calafat. 2004. Urinary levels of seven phthalate metabolites in the U.S. population from the National Health and Nutrition Examination Survey (NHANES) 1999-2000. Environ. Health Perspect. 112(3):331-338.

Skakkebæk, N.E., E. Rajpert-De Meyts, and K.M. Main. 2001. Testicular dysgenesis syndrome: An increasingly common developmental disorder with environmental aspects. Hum. Reprod. 16(5): 972-978.

Van den Berg, M., L.S. Birnbaum, M. Denison, M. De Vito, W. Farland, M. Feeley, H. Fiedler, H. Hakansson, A. Hanberg, L. Haws, M. Rose, S. Safe, D. Schrenk, C. Tohyama, A. Tritscher, J. Tuomisto, M. Tysklind, N. Walker, and R.E. Peterson. 2006. The 2005 World Health Organization reevaluation of human and mammalian toxic equivalency factors for dioxins and dioxin-like compounds. Toxicol. Sci. 93(2):223-241.

2

Phthalate Exposure Assessment in Humans

As mentioned in Chapter 1, phthalates[1] are chemicals used as plasticizers in polymers to impart flexibility and durability to a multitude of everyday products and for their solvent properties in other products. Phthalates may be classified into two groups based on molecular weight. Accordingly, low-molecular-weight phthalates (ester side-chain lengths, one to four carbons) include DMP, DEP, DBP, and DIBP, and high-molecular-weight phthalates (ester side-chain lengths, five or more carbons) include DEHP, DOP, and DINP.

This chapter briefly describes what is known about phthalate exposures in humans and includes an overview of important sources and routes of exposures; some human exposure levels, including those of susceptible or highly exposed populations; and metabolism and pharmacokinetics. Many questions remain unanswered about cumulative exposures to phthalates throughout the life span, relative contributions of various sources of exposure to the phthalate body burden over time, and mixed exposures that may include phthalates or other chemicals that may elicit common adverse outcomes. Despite those limitations, the existing information on human exposure to phthalates can be used to help determine whether cumulative risk assessment should be conducted for phthalates. This chapter provides the context for the discussion of cumulative risk assessment and is not meant to be a quantitative exposure assessment of any particular phthalate or the chemical class as a whole.

PHTHALATE SOURCES AND ROUTES OF EXPOSURE

Phthalates used as plasticizers in polymers are not chemically bound to the polymers and therefore readily leach, migrate, or off-gas from the polymers, particularly when phthalate-containing products are exposed to high tempera-

---

[1]As stated in Chapter 1, the term *phthalates* used in this report refers to diesters of 1,2-benzenedicarboxylic acid, the *o*-phthalates.

tures. Low-molecular-weight phthalates—including DMP, DEP, and DBP—are used in a variety of personal-hygiene and cosmetic products, such as nail polish to minimize chipping and fragrances as scent stabilizers (ATSDR 1995, 2001; NICNAC 2008). High-molecular-weight phthalates—including DEHP, DINP, and DOP—are used in plastic tubing, food packaging and processing materials, containers, vinyl toys, vinyl floor coverings, and building products (ATSDR 1997, 2002; ECB 2003; Kueseng et al. 2007). Medical supplies and devices may contain phthalates, as may some medications (for example, medications with enteric coatings) (Hauser et al. 2004). Table 2-1 lists some common phthalates and examples of their uses.

Phthalate exposures may occur through ingestion, inhalation, dermal absorption, and parenteral administration. The relative contributions of the exposures to the total body burden at various ages are not known.

BIOMARKERS OF EXPOSURE

Both animal and human studies demonstrate that exposure may occur throughout the life span, from the developing fetus through early infancy, childhood, and beyond. Phthalates can cross the placenta (Saillenfait et al. 1998; Fennell et al. 2004), have been measured in amniotic fluid in human studies (Silva et al. 2004), are present in breast milk (Parmar et al. 1985; Dostal et al. 1987), and can be measured in urine at all ages (CDC 2003, 2005; Sathyanarayana et al. 2008).

Human exposure to phthalates is assessed most frequently by measuring urinary polar metabolites. Urinary excretion of polar molecules is efficient, and their urinary concentration is generally 5-20 times that in lipid-rich body compartments. For example, the urinary concentrations of MEHP, MIBP, MEP, and MBP were 20-100 times those in blood or milk (Högberg et al. 2008). Recent advances in urinary phthalate biomarkers have led to the measurement of the oxidized metabolites; measuring these metabolites eliminates the potential problems of contamination inherent in measuring the parent compounds and their monoesters. The utility of other biologic matrices—such as blood, breast milk, and seminal plasma—for assessing human exposure remains largely unknown because there are few data. The incorporation of those novel matrices into human studies necessitates the measurement of oxidized metabolites to avoid problems with contamination by the ubiquitous parent diesters.

Exposure of the U.S. and German population to at least 10 phthalates has been demonstrated by measurement of their urinary metabolites as shown in Table 2-2. Other reports generally have found exposures similar to or consistent with those in Table 2-2 with respect to age, sex, and racial or ethnic variations. Except for MEP, urinary metabolites in U.S. children, males, Hispanics, and blacks are generally somewhat higher than those in adults shown in Table 2-2 (CDC 2005).

TABLE 2-1 Common Phthalates and Examples of Uses

Phthalate	Uses
DMP	Insect repellent, plastic
DEP	Shampoo, scents, soap, lotion, cosmetics, industrial solvent, medications
DBP	Adhesives, caulk, cosmetics, industrial solvent, medications
DIBP	Adhesives, caulk, cosmetics, industrial solvent
BBP	Vinyl flooring, adhesives, sealants, industrial solvent
DCHP	Stabilizer in rubber, polymers
DEHP	Soft plastic, including tubing, toys, home products, food containers, food packaging
DOP	Soft plastic
DINP	Soft plastics, replacement for DEHP

In Germany, concentrations of MBP and of DEHP metabolites decreased over the period 1988-2003 (Wittassek et al. 2007). In the United States, MBP concentrations also decreased over the period 1999-2002; however, no decline was noted for MEHP (CDC 2003, 2005). Data released by the National Health and Nutrition Examination Survey (NHANES) demonstrate exposure to multiple phthalates in most people (CDC 2003, 2005). Data from Wittassek et al. (2007) and Sathyanarayana et al. (2008) also indicate exposure to multiple phthalates.

Infant and Childhood Exposure

NHANES data show that concentrations of urinary phthalate metabolites in children 6-11 years old were higher than those in adolescents and adults (CDC 2005). Several studies support the Centers for Disease Control and Prevention's findings that children have higher urinary concentrations than adults of DBP, BBP, and DEHP (Brock et al. 2002; Koch et al. 2004, 2005a). Differences between children and adults in the amount of urine produced per unit body weight and in body surface area may contribute to differences in urinary concentrations of specific metabolites. Whether the observed differences in urinary concentrations between children and adults result from differences in exposure or metabolism or both is unclear. In a recent study (Sathyanarayana et al. 2008), urine samples from infants were found to have detectable concentrations of multiple urinary phthalate metabolites, which suggested that exposure to multiple phthalates is common even early in life. Studies of urine samples of pregnant women (Adibi et al. 2008; Wolff et al. 2008) have suggested that fetuses may also be exposed to multiple phthalates.

TABLE 2-2 Urinary Phthalate Metabolites in Large Studies in United States and Germany

Concentration, µg/L[a]

Parent Compound	Metabolite	CDC 2005 NHANES, United States 2001-2002 Spot Urine Sample N = 1,647, over 20 y old		Wittassek et al. 2007 Germany 1988-2003 24-h Urine Sample N = 634, 20-29 y old		Silva et al. 2007a United States 2003-2004 Spot Urine Sample N = 129, Adults	
		50th %	95th %	50th %	95th %	50th %	95th %
DMP	MMP	1.40	9.10	–	–	–	–
DEP	MEP	181	2,720	–	–	–	–
DBP	MBP	19.1	95.4	112	604	–	–
DIBP	MIBP	2.4	16.3	34.5	176	–	–
BBP	MBZP	13.8	99.7	7.4	50.4	–	–
DCHP	MCHP	<LOD	0.500	–	–	–	–
DEHP	MECPP	–	–	26.9	98.8	–	–
	MEHHP	17.7	175	21.0	77.2	–	–
	MEOHP	12.2	115	16.7	57.5	–	–
	MEHP	4.10	39.5	7.6	33.6	–	–
DOP	MCPP	2.60	12.0	–	–	–	–
	MOP	<LOD	<LOD	–	–	–	–
DINP	MINP	<LOD	<LOD	–	–	–	–
	MHINP	–	–	2.0	11.9	–	–
	MOINP	–	–	1.0	5.6	–	–

DIDP						
MCINP	—	—	—	—	4.4	104.4
MHIDP	—	—	—	—	4.9	70.6
MOIDP	—	—	—	—	1.2	15.0
MIDP	—	—	—	—	<LOD	<LOD

[a] —, data not obtained; LOD, limit of detection.

Note: LODs vary by study and by analyte but are generally less than 1 μg/L.

Several factors are unique to infants and children and may affect exposure to multiple phthalates. Differences in urinary concentrations of phthalates among infants, children, and adults may reflect different sources and routes of intake. Ingestion is thought to be a primary pathway of exposure to some phthalates, especially those in food packaging (Shea et al. 2003; Kueseng et al. 2007). Infants and young children consume more calories per kilogram of body weight and consume relatively more dairy and other fatty foods, such as milk and infant formulas, which have been found to contain phthalates (Sorensen 2006). Infants and toddlers also demonstrate age-appropriate mouthing behaviors that potentially increase their exposures to phthalates in children's toys and other products made with plasticized polymers.

Indoor air is another source of exposure to phthalates from a variety of sources, including aerosols generated from polyvinyl chloride household products, such as vinyl flooring and shower curtains, and indoor deodorants (Adibi et al. 2003; Rudel et al. 2003). Infants and young children have higher specific respiratory rates than adults (Etzel and Balk 2003; EPA 2006) and thus have potentially higher specific exposures via inhalation.

In summary, infants' and children's physiology, developmental stages, and age-appropriate behaviors all may increase exposure to phthalates. Consequently, they may be especially vulnerable to phthalate exposures during critical stages of growth and development.

Highly Exposed Populations

Highly exposed people have urinary metabolite concentrations that often exceed those at the 95th percentile of the general population (Table 2-3). Widely recognized as potentially highly exposed are neonates receiving medical treatments, such as transfusions (Shea et al. 2003; Green et al. 2005). Neonates in the intensive care unit experience high exposures because many medical devices are made of polyvinyl chloride plastics that may contain phthalates (Sjoberg et al. 1985; Green et al. 2005); thus, for neonates and others using parenteral devices, this is another important route to consider. Some medications contain phthalates in their coatings or delivery systems (Hauser et al. 2005) and may contribute to high exposures of children, pregnant women, and others taking these medications.

METABOLISM, PHARMACOKINETICS, AND IMPLICATIONS FOR POSSIBLE SUSCEPTIBILITY

Mammalian absorption and metabolism of phthalates (see Figure 2-1) are rapid; initial de-esterification of one alkyl linkage occurs in the saliva or the gut after oral intake. The resulting monoesters have one carboxylic acid and one

TABLE 2-3 Urinary Phthalate Metabolite Concentrations after Exceptional Exposures and Comparison Medians from Available NHANES or European Union Data

Exposure	Metabolite Concentrations in Urine (µg/L)	NHANES or EU Medians [95th %] (µg/L)	Reference
Enteric-coated medication taken orally for 3 mo (n = 1 male)	MBP 16,868 MEP 444 MEHP 3 MBZP 9	MBP 19.3 [95][a] MEP 171 [3,050][a] MEHP 4.3 [38][a] MBZP 16 [122][a]	Hauser et al. 2004
Intravenous tubing for platelet donation, maximum measured 4 h after donation (n = 1 male)	MEHP 388 MEHHP 822 MEOHP 729 MECPP 577	MEHP 7.6 [34][b] MEHHP 21 [77][b] MEOHP 16.7 [58][b] MECPP 26.9 [99][b]	Koch et al. 2005b
Neonatal intensive care unit, 33 samples from infants exposed for over 2 wk (n = 6)	MEHP 129[c] MEHHP 2,221[c] MEOHP 1,697[c]	MEHP 4.4 [30][d] MEHHP 32.9 [210][d] MEOHP 22.6 [142][d]	Calafat et al. 2004
Infants in neonatal intensive care unit (n = 54)	MEHP 22 (75th % = 71)[c] MEHHP 267 (75th % = 644)[c] MEOHP 256 (75th % = 628)[c] MBP 18 (75th % = 45)[c] MBZP 41 (75th % = 131)[c]	MEHP 4.4 [30][d] MEHHP 32.9 [210][d] MEOHP 22.6 [142][d] MBP 32.4 [157][d] MBZP 37 [226][d]	Weuve et al. 2006
Plastisol workers after shift (n = 25)	MEHP 56[e] MECPP 104[e]	MEHP 4.3 [38][a]	Gaudin et al. 2008

[a]U.S. males over 25 years old from NHANES 2001-2002 (CDC 2005).
[b]German adults 20-29 years old (Wittassek et al. 2007).
[c]Median values, unless otherwise stated.
[d]U.S. children 6-11 years old from NHANES 2001-2002 (CDC 2005). No data are available on neonates.
[e]Medians before shift, 16 µg/L (MEHP) and 38 µg/L (MECPP), which were slightly higher than in controls.

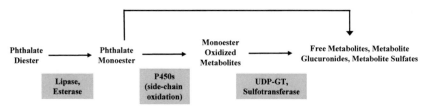

FIGURE 2-1 Phthalate metabolism. UDP-GT, uridine 5'-diphosphate-glucuronosyltransferase.

ester substituent with a side chain of one or more carbons. Monoesters are the main detected metabolites of the low-molecular-weight phthalates, such as DEP and DBP (Silva et al. 2007b; Wittassek and Angerer 2008). However, phthalate monoesters with five or more carbons in the ester side chain (for example, MEHP, MOP, and MNP) are efficiently transformed further to oxidized metabolites arising mainly from ω-oxidation at the terminal or penultimate carbon of the alkyl ester side chain (for example, MECCP and MEOHP for DEHP; see Figure 2-2). For esters with side chains of five or more carbons, the oxidized metabolites are the primary metabolites found in urine. The proportions of numerous oxidized metabolites vary among parent phthalates (see Table 1-1). The first-round ω-oxidation products dominate for MEHP, but MOP and MNP can lose additional two-carbon units sequentially via ß-oxidation at the ester terminal side chain. Thus, the longer the alkyl side chain, the greater variety of oxidized metabolites (Wittassek and Angerer 2008). As a result, little monoester from the high-molecular-weight phthalates is detected, typically less than 10% of the absorbed dose (Barr et al. 2003; Koch et al. 2003).

Monoesters and oxidized metabolites are excreted free or conjugated as glucuronides—and to a small extent sulfates—and mainly in urine (Silva et al. 2003; Kato et al. 2004; CDC 2005; Calafat et al. 2006; Silva et al. 2007a). However, the low-molecular-weight phthalate metabolites, such as MEP and MBP, are eliminated quickly, yielding a large proportion of the free nonpolar monoesters, whereas the more polar oxidized metabolites have a greater proportion of conjugated monoesters (Silva et al. 2006). For most phthalates, urinary monoester concentrations may not constitute a major fraction of absorbed dose. For example, the primary metabolite of DBP is MBP (about 90%), whereas less than 10% of metabolites of long-chain phthalates are monoesters. Specifically, MECPP is the primary metabolite of DEHP (greater than 25%), MHINP is the primary DINP metabolite (greater than 20%), and MHPHP is the primary DPHP metabolite (greater than 15%) (Wittassek and Angerer 2008). Therefore, human exposure to the low-molecular-weight phthalates can be adequately assessed with urinary monoesters, but exposure to the high-molecular-weight phthalates, such as DEHP and DINP, have been underestimated by measuring only monoesters and failing to account for other metabolites.

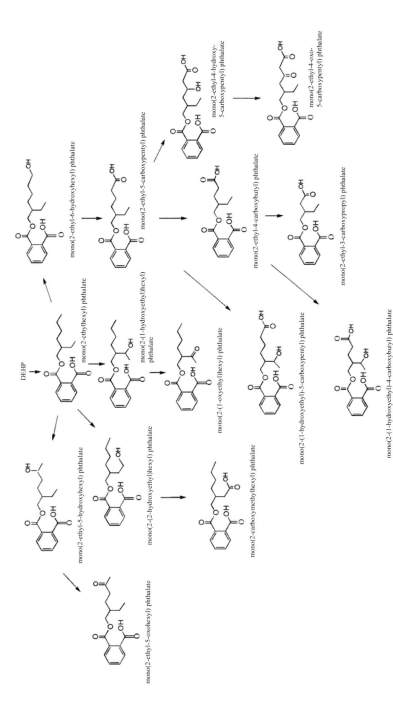

FIGURE 2-2 DEHP metabolism. Source: Adapted from Silva et al. 2006. Reprinted with permission; copyright 2006, *Toxicology*.

Oxidized metabolites have several important advantages as biomarkers of exposure. First, phthalates are ubiquitous in the environment. They often contaminate biospecimens, becoming precursors of monoesters that can be formed by endogenous esterases (as in serum in a vacutainer) or by chemical hydrolysis or photolysis during the course of sample collection, storage, and analysis. In contrast, the oxidized metabolites can be formed in vivo only from the monoester and only via hepatic metabolism; therefore, they do not arise from external contamination. A second advantage is that they have longer half-lives than the monoesters, which are either rapidly excreted or quickly oxidized. Accordingly, the oxidized metabolites may be more reflective of average exposure than the rapidly excreted monoesters, at least in the case of phthalates with ester side chains of five or more carbons.

The complex pharmacokinetics of various phthalates may have implications for toxicity in that some metabolites have more potent biologic activity than others. For example, the monoesters are thought to be those most relevant to androgen insufficiency (Shono et al. 2000; Kai et al. 2005). Therefore, exposure-assessment strategies aimed at risk assessment may need to choose whether to focus on specific metabolites or on the total body burden as reflecting exposure to the parent phthalates.

There are as yet unexplained interindividual differences in metabolic capacity at each step of phthalate metabolism, which may account for some of the differences seen in urinary metabolites by age, sex, race, and other demographic factors. Such differences may explain the observation that the urinary concentrations of oxidized metabolites are more prevalent in children than in adults (Koch et al. 2004; CDC 2005; Koch et al. 2005a). Neonates show a striking difference, with urinary MECPP concentrations being higher proportionally than in older subjects (Koch et al. 2006). Conversely, the lack of oxidized metabolites in amniotic fluid might be explained by immature expression of some enzymes, such as esterases, and oxidation, glucuronidation, and sulfation enzymes by fetuses. At this time, however, it is not known which specific enzymes are involved in phthalate metabolism in humans (McCarver and Hines 2002; Shea et al. 2003; Blake et al. 2005). Differences in metabolism may have potential implications for risk. Therefore, improved knowledge concerning the biologic basis of variability in exposure related to age, race, sex, and other factors may provide a better understanding of differences in susceptibility to phthalate toxicity.

PHARMACOKINETIC MODELS OF PHTHALATES

The phthalates on which pharmacokinetic data are most extensive are DBP and DEHP. Human absorption of phthalates is efficient after oral exposure and can occur after dermal exposure (Koch et al. 2006; Janjua et al. 2007). Evidence is sparser with respect to respiratory intake. Adibi et al. (2008) reported positive correlations between air measurements of BBP, DIBP, and DEP and urinary concentrations of MBZP, MIBP, and MEP, respectively, but Becker et al. (2004)

did not find a correlation between DEHP in house dust and urinary concentrations of DEHP metabolites. Phthalate metabolism is qualitatively similar among species, beginning with formation of the monoester, which can be excreted unchanged, glucuronidated, sulfated, or further oxidized (Albro et al. 1984; Pollack et al. 1985a,b; Koch et al. 2006; Clewell et al. 2008). However, the rates of metabolism and proportions of the various metabolites vary by species and by diester structure, especially the length and saturation of the alkyl side chain of the diester as described above.

Physiologically based pharmacokinetic (PBPK) models have been developed for the two better studied phthalates, DBP and DEHP. Keys et al. (1999, 2000) first developed PBPK models to evaluate the role of various transport processes in the clearance of MBP and MEHP in the adult male rat. The models accurately describe plasma MBP and MEHP kinetics after administration of the phthalates. More recently, a PBPK model was developed for disposition of DBP in the adult, pregnant, and fetal rat (Clewell et al. 2008). This model describes the time course of urinary, plasma, bile, and fecal clearance of DBP, MBP (the biologically active metabolite), and the glucuronide and oxidized metabolites after single (oral or intravenous) or repeated (oral) DBP exposures at 1-500 mg/kg. With the model, it is possible to estimate fetal MBP exposure from other exposure metrics, including external dose, maternal plasma and urine, and amniotic fluid. Thus, the model provides a means of extrapolating rat fetal dose from different phthalate exposure biomarkers in various compartments or biologic matrices. The DBP model has also been extrapolated for use in the human by adjusting the physiologic parameters and scaling chemical-specific parameters allometrically. Preliminary results reported in an abstract (Campbell et al. 2007) indicated that the model was able to predict MBP concentrations in the urine of human adults given controlled doses of DBP without changing chemical-specific parameters; this suggested that the metabolism of DBP to MBP and of MBP to MBP-glucuronide is similar in the rat and human at human-relevant doses. In particular, the kinetics of free MBP and MBP-glucuronide are well described by the allometric scaling.

The DBP gestation model has also been applied to DEHP, a phthalate with different kinetics from DBP (Clewell et al., 2007). In vitro data and in vivo observations were used to adjust the chemical-specific model parameters, and data on plasma, tissue, and excreta MEHP concentrations in the adult, pregnant, and fetal rat after DEHP administration (Kessler et al. 2004) were used to test the model.

The predictive models can be evaluated by using cross-sectional data on rats and humans, which allow a crude comparison of phthalate exposure biomarkers in amniotic fluid, urine, and maternal and fetal serum. The data suggest that concentrations in maternal and fetal serum are similar to those in amniotic fluid, and all three compartments have lower concentrations than those in urine (Silva et al. 2004; Calafat et al. 2006; Silva et al. 2007b). The estimates are similar to those in reports of other polar environmental biomarkers in amniotic fluid, urine, and blood (Engel et al. 2006; Foster et al. 2002; CDC 2005)

The findings on DBP and DEHP from experimental pharmacokinetic models in various life stages and species based on known physiologic differences, although relying on few data, suggest that the approach may also be useful for describing the disposition of other phthalates in the rat and human. Such information on disposition is needed for both quantitative and qualitative evaluation of the array of human phthalate exposures. Future goals should include development of models that can provide reasonable estimates of the concentrations of "active phthalates" in the fetus or mother after mixed exposures.

AMNIOTIC FLUID: THE FETAL COMPARTMENT

Amniotic fluid can be used to estimate fetal exposure and consists largely of fetal urine, especially late in gestation (Gabbe et al. 2007). There is only one published study on phthalate metabolites in human amniotic fluid, which is based on 54 anonymously collected samples. Amniotic fluid concentrations of MEP, MBP, and MEHP exceeded the limit of detection in 93%, 39%, and 24% of samples, respectively (Silva et al. 2004). MBZP was detected in only one sample. The oxidized DEHP metabolites MEHHP and MEOHP, which are usually found in higher concentrations than MEHP in maternal urine (Barr et al. 2003), were not detected in amniotic fluid. Similarly, in rats, free MEHP and MBP were the predominant metabolites in amniotic fluid (Calafat et al. 2006), but oxidized metabolites were not measured.

Paired urine samples from the women providing amniotic fluid samples were not available. Nevertheless, the concentrations of MEP, MBP, and MEHP in amniotic fluid were generally lower than median urinary concentrations from NHANES 1999-2000 (NCHS 2008). Because uridine diphosphate glucuronosyltransferase isoenzymes are not fully expressed until after birth (Coughtrie et al. 1988; de Wildt et al. 1999), the fetus may be unable to glucuronidate the phthalate monoesters; in turn, clearance from the fetal compartment may be slower.

The lack of detectable DEHP oxidized metabolites in the human amniotic fluid samples (no measurements were made in the rat study) raises several intriguing issues. It may indicate that the fetus is unable to oxidatively metabolize MEHP because of immature P450 enzymes. Alternatively, the presence of MEHP without the oxidized metabolites may indicate contamination of the amniotic fluid with DEHP during collection or storage and then hydrolysis to MEHP in the amniotic fluid. Alternatively, it is possible that passive transfer of maternal oxidized metabolites across the placental barrier is not efficient or that they are excreted so rapidly that the resulting low serum concentrations lead to little transfer. Indeed, rat studies suggest that maternal DEHP dose is correlated with urinary and amniotic fluid concentrations of MEHP and MEHHP but that relationships are not linear (Calafat et al. 2006). Because it is difficult—and not generally possible—to obtain amniotic fluid, apart from clinical procedures or at delivery, there is a need for human studies to determine metabolite concentrations and understand the relationship between metabolite concentrations in amniotic fluid and maternal urine samples. Two recent reports (Adibi et al. 2008; Wolff et al. 2008) indicate that the urinary concentrations of phthalates in pregnant women are consistent with the previously published NHANES data on women of reproductive age.

CONCLUSIONS

Our understanding of important sources of, routes of exposure to, and metabolism of phthalates in humans has increased over the last decade. Recent data have shown widespread human exposure to multiple phthalates from a multitude of sources. Studies have also identified high-exposure groups that may be more vulnerable to the effects of phthalates and their metabolites. Those groups potentially include the fetus and child, whose exposure and metabolism may differ from those of the adult and impart differences in risk. Despite our increased understanding, important unresolved issues remain; research needs are described in Chapter 6 of this report.

REFERENCES

Adibi, J.J., F.P. Perera, W. Jedrychowski, D.E. Camann, D. Barr, R. Jacek, and R.M. Whyatt. 2003. Prenatal exposures to phthalates among women in New York City and Krakow, Poland. Environ. Health Perspect. 111(14):1719-1722.

Adibi, J.J., R.M. Whyatt, P.L. Williams, A.M. Calafat, D. Camann, R. Herrick, H. Nelson, H.K. Bhat, F.P. Perera, M.J. Silva, and R. Hauser. 2008. Characterization of phthalate exposure among pregnant women assessed by repeat air and urine samples. Environ. Health Perspect. 116(4):467-473.

Albro, P.W., K. Chae, R. Philpot, J.T. Corbett, J. Schroeder, and S. Jordan. 1984. In vitro metabolism of mono-2-ethylhexyl phthalate by microsomal enzymes. Similarity to omega- and (omega-1) oxidation of fatty acids. Drug Metab. Dispos. 12(6):742-748.

ATSDR (Agency for Toxic Substances and Disease Registry). 1995. Toxicological Profile for Diethyl Phthalate. U.S. Department of Health and Human Services, Public Health Service, Agency for Toxic Substances and Disease Registry, Atlanta, GA. June 1995 [online]. Available: http://www.atsdr.cdc.gov/toxprofiles/tp73.pdf [accessed Sept. 22, 2008].

ATSDR (Agency for Toxic Substances and Disease Registry). 1997. Toxicological Profile for Di-n-Octylphthalate. U.S. Department of Health and Human Services, Public Health Service, Agency for Toxic Substances and Disease Registry, Atlanta, GA. September 1997 [online]. Available: http://www.atsdr.cdc.gov/toxprofiles/tp95.pdf [accessed Sept. 22, 2008].

ATSDR (Agency for Toxic Substances and Disease Registry). 2001. Toxicological Profile for Di-n-Butyl Phthalate. U.S. Department of Health and Human Services, Public Health Service, Agency for Toxic Substances and Disease Registry, Atlanta, GA. September 2001 [online]. Available: http://www.atsdr.cdc.gov/toxprofiles/tp135.pdf [accessed Sept. 22, 2008].

ATSDR (Agency for Toxic Substances and Disease Registry). 2002. Toxicological Profile for Di(2-ethylhexyl)phthalate. U.S. Department of Health and Human Services, Public Health Service, Agency for Toxic Substances and Disease Registry, Atlanta, GA. September 2002 [online]. Available: http://www.atsdr.cdc.gov/tox profiles/tp9.pdf [accessed Sept. 22, 2008].

Barr, D.B., M.J. Silva, K. Kato, J.A. Reidy, N.A. Malek, D. Hurtz, M. Sadowski, L.L. Needham, and A.M Calafat. 2003. Assessing human exposure to phthalates using monoesters and their oxidized metabolites as biomarkers. Environ. Health Perspect. 111(9):1148-1151.

Becker, K., M. Seiwert, J. Angerer, W. Heger, H.M. Koch, R. Nagorka, E. Rosskamp, C. Schlüter, B. Seifert, and D. Ullrich. 2004. DEHP metabolites in urine of children and DEHP in house dust. Int. J. Hyg. Environ. Health 207(5):409-417.

Blake, M.J., L. Castro, J.S. Leeder, and G.L. Kearns. 2005. Ontogeny of drug metabolizing enzymes in the neonate. Semin. Fetal Neonatal Med. 10(2):123-138.

Brock, J.W., S.P. Caudill, M.J. Silva, L.L. Needham, and E.D. Hilborn. 2002. Phthalate monoesters levels in the urine of young children. Bull. Environ. Contam. Toxicol. 6(3):309-314.

Calafat, A.M., L.L. Needham, M.J. Silva, and G. Lambert. 2004. Exposure to di-(2-ethylhexyl) phthalate among premature neonates in a neonatal intensive care unit. Pediatrics 113(5):e429-434.

Calafat, A.M., J.W. Brock, M.J. Silva, L.E. Gray Jr., J.A. Reidy, D.B. Barr, and L.L. Needham. 2006. Urinary and amniotic fluid levels of phthalate monoesters in rats after the oral administration of di(2-ethylhexyl) phthalate and di-n-butyl phthalate. Toxicology 217(1):22-30.

Campbell, J.L., Jr., Y.M. Tan, R.A. Clewell, and H.J. Clewell III. 2007. Physiologically Based Pharmacokinetic Model for Monobutyl Phthalate: Interpreting Biomonitoring Data to Assess Human Exposure and Risk. Abstract M4-D4. Presented at the Society for Risk Analysis Annual Meeting 2007-Risk 007: Agents of Analysis, December 9-12, 2007, San Antonio, TX [online]. Available: http://birenheide.com/sra/2007AM/program/singlesession.php3?sessid=M4-D [accessed July 15, 2008].

CDC (Centers for Disease Control and Prevention). 2003. Second National Report on Human Exposure to Environmental Chemicals. NCEH Pub. No. 02-0716. U.S. Department of Health and Human Services, Centers for Disease Control and Prevention, Atlanta GA. January 2003 [online]. Available: http://www.jhsph.edu/ephtcenter/Second%20Report.pdf [accessed Sept. 22, 2008].

CDC (Centers for Disease Control and Prevention). 2005. Third National Report on Human Exposure to Environmental Chemicals. NCEH Pub. No. 05-0570. National Center for Environmental Health Division of Laboratory Sciences, Centers for Disease Control and Prevention, Atlanta, GA [online]. Available: http://www.cdc.gov/exposurereport/report.htm [accessed July 15, 2008].

Clewell, R.A., S.J. Borghoff, and M.E. Andersen. 2007. Application of a unified PBPK model to two kinetically distinct phthalate esters - DBP and DEHP. Toxicologist. 96(1):348 [Abstract 1682].

Clewell, R.A, J.J. Kremer, C.C. Williams, J.L. Campbell Jr., M.E. Andersen, and S.J. Borghoff. 2008. Tissue exposures to free and glucuronidated monobutylphthalate in the pregnant and fetal rat following exposure to di-n-butylphthalate: Evaluation with a PBPK model. Toxicol. Sci. 103(2): 241-259.

Coughtrie, M.W., B. Burchell, J.E. Leakey, and R. Hume. 1988. The inadequacy of perinatal glucuonidation: Immunoblot analysis of the developmental expression of individual UDP-glucuronosyltransferase isoenzymes in rat and human liver microsomes. Mol. Pharmacol. 34(6):729-735.

de Wildt, S.N., G.L. Kearns, J.S. Leeder, and J.N. van den Anker. 1999. Glucuronidation in humans. Pharmacogenetic and developmental aspects. Clin. Pharmacokinet. 36(6):439-452.

Dostal, L.A., R.P. Weaver, and B.A. Schwetz. 1987. Transfer of di(2ethylhexyl)phthalate through rat milk and effects on milk consumption and the mammary gland. Toxicol. Appl. Pharmacol. 91(3):315-325.

ECB (European Chemicals Bureau). 2003. European Union Risk Assessment Report: 1,2-benzenedicarboxyl Acid, Di-C8-10-branched Alkyl Esters, C9-rich and Di-"Isononyl" Phthalate (DINP)CAS Nos: 68515-48-0 and 28553-12-0; EINECS Nos: 271-090-9 and 249-079-5, S.J. Munn, R. Allanou, K. Aschberger, F. Berthault, J. de Bruijn, C. Musset, S. O'Connor, S. Pakalin, G. Pellegrini, S. Scheer, and S. Vegro, eds. EUR 20784EN. Luxembourg: Office for Official Publications of the European Communities [online]. Available: http://ecb.jrc.ec. europa.eu/documents/Existing-Chemicals/RISK_ASSESSMENT/REPORT/dinpre port046.pdf [accessed Sept. 22, 2008].

Engel, S.M., B. Levy, Z. Liu, D. Kaplan, and M.S. Wolff. 2006. Xenobiotic phenols in early pregnancy amniotic fluid. Reprod. Toxicol. 21(1):110-112.

EPA (U.S. Environmental Protection Agency). 2006. Metabolically-Derived Human Ventilation Rates: A Revised Approach Based Upon Oxygen Consumption Rates. External Review Draft. EPA/600/R-06/129A. National Center for Environmental Assessment, Office of Research and Development, U.S. Environmental Protection Agency, Washington, DC. October 31, 2006 [online]. Available: http://cfpub.epa. gov/ncea/cfm/recordisplay.cfm?deid=160065 [accessed July 15, 2008].

Etzel, R.A., and S.J. Balk, eds. 2003. Handbook of Pediatric Environmental Health, 2nd Ed. Elk Grove Village, IL: American Academy of Pediatrics.

Fennell, T.R., W.L. Krol, S.C. Sumner, and R.W. Snyder. 2004. Pharmacokinetics of dibutylphthalate in pregnant rats. Toxicol. Sci. 82(2):407-418.

Foster, W.G., S. Chan, L. Platt, and C.L. Hughes, Jr. 2002. Detection of phytoestrogens in samples of second trimester human amniotic fluid. Toxicol. Lett. 129(3):199-205.

Gabbe, S.G., J.L. Simpson, J.R. Niebyl, H. Galan, L. Goetzl, E.R.M. Jauniaux, and M. Landon. 2007. Obstetrics: Normal and Problem Pregnancies, 5th Ed. Philadelphia: Churchill Livingstone/Elsevier.

Gaudin, R., P. Marsan, A. Robert, P. Ducos, A. Pruvost, M. Levi, and P. Bouscaillou. 2008. Biological monitoring of occupational exposure to di(2-ethylhexyl) phthalate: Survey of workers exposed to plastisols. Int. Arch. Occup. Environ. Health 81(8):959-966.

Green, R., R. Hauser, A.M. Calafat, J. Weuve, T. Schettler, S. Ringer, K. Huttner, and H. Hu. 2005. Use of di(2-ethylhexyl) phthalate-containing medical products and urinary levels of mono(2-ethylhexyl) phthalate in neonatal intensive care unit infants. Environ. Health Perspect. 113(9):1222-1225.

Hauser, R., S. Duty, L. Godfrey-Bailey, and A.M. Calafat. 2004. Medications as a source of human exposure to phthalates. Environ. Health Perspect. 112(6):751-753.

Hauser, R., P. Williams, L. Altshul, and A.M. Calafat. 2005. Evidence of interaction between polychlorinated biphenyls and phthalates in relation to human sperm motility. Environ. Health Perspect. 113(4):425-430.

Högberg, J., A. Hanberg, M. Berglund, S. Skerfving, M. Remberger, A.M. Calafat, A.F. Filipsson, B. Jansson, N. Johansson, M. Appelgren, and H. Hakansson. 2008. Phthalate diesters and their metabolites in human breast milk, blood or serum, and urine as biomarkers of exposure in vulnerable populations. Environ. Health Perspect. 116(3):334-339.

Janjua, N.R., G.K. Mortensen, A.M. Andersson, B. Kongshoj, N.E. Skakkebæk, and H.C. Wulf. 2007. Systemic uptake of diethyl phthalate, dibutyl phthalate, and butyl paraben following whole-body topical application and reproductive and thyroid hormone levels in humans. Environ. Sci. Technol. 41(15):5564-5570.

Kai, H., T. Shono, T. Tajiri, and S. Suita. 2005. Long-term effects of intrauterine exposure to mono-n-butyl phthalate on the reproductive function of postnatal rats. J. Pediatr. Surg. 40(2):429-433.

Kato, K., M.J. Silva, J.A. Reidy, D. Hurtz, N.A. Malek, L.L. Needham, H. Nakazawa, D.B. Barr, and A.M. Calafat. 2004. Mono(2-ethyl-5-hydroxyhexyl) phthalate and mono-(2-ethyl-5-oxohexyl) phthalate as biomarkers for human exposure assessment to di-(2-ethylhexyl) phthalate. Environ. Health Perspect. 112(3):327-330.

Kessler, W., W. Numtip, K. Grote, G.A. Csanády, I. Chahoud, and J.G. Filser. 2004. Blood burden of di(2-ethylhexyl) phthalate and its primary metabolite mono(2-ethylhexyl) phthalate in pregnant and nonpregnant rats and marmosets. Toxicol. Appl. Pharmacol. 195(2):142-153.

Keys, D.A., D.G. Wallace, T.B. Kepler, and R.B. Conolly. 1999. Quantitative evaluation of alternative mechanisms of blood and testes disposition of di(2-ethylhexyl) phthalate and mono(2-ethylhexyl) phthalate in rats. Toxicol. Sci. 49(2):172-185.

Keys, D.A., D.G. Wallace, T.B. Kepler, and R.B. Conolly. 2000. Quantitative evaluation of alternative mechanisms of blood disposition of di(n-butyl) phthalate and mono(n-butyl) phthalate in rats. Toxicol. Sci. 53(2):173-184.

Koch, H.M., B. Rossbach, H. Drexler, and J. Angerer. 2003. Internal exposure of the general population to DEHP and other phthalates—determination of secondary and primary phthalate monoester metabolites in urine. Environ. Res. 93(2):177-185.

Koch, H.M., H. Drexler, and J. Angerer. 2004. Internal exposure of nursery-school children and their parents and teachers to di(2-ethylhexyl) phthalate (DEHP). Int. J. Hyg. Environ. Health 207(1):15-22.

Koch, H.M., R. Preuss, H. Drexeler, and J. Angerer. 2005a. Exposure of nursery school children and their parents and teachers to di-n-butylphthalate and butylbenzylphthalate. Int. Arch. Occup. Environ. Health 78(3):223-229.

Koch, H.M., H.M. Bolt, R. Preuss, R. Eckstein, V. Weisbach, and J. Angerer. 2005b. Intravenous exposure to di(2-ethylhexyl) phthalate (DEHP): Metabolites of DEHP in urine after a voluntary platelet donation. Arch. Toxicol. 79(12):689-693.

Koch, H.M., R. Preuss, and J. Angerer. 2006. Di(2-ethylhexyl) phthalate (DEHP): Human metabolism and internal exposure—an update and latest results. Int. J. Androl. 29(1):155-165.

Kueseng, P., P. Thavarungkul, and P. Kanatharana. 2007. Trace phthalate and adipate esters contaminated in packaged food. J. Environ. Sci. Health 42(5):569-576.

McCarver, D.G., and R.H. Hines. 2002. The ontogeny of human drug-metabolizing enzymes: Phase II conjugation enzymes and regulatory mechanisms. J. Pharmacol. Exp. Ther. 300(2):361-366.

NCHS (National Center for Health Statistics). 2008. National Health and Nutrition Examination Survey: Data Sets and Related Documentation. U.S. Department of Health and Human Services, Centers for Disease Control and Prevention, National Center for Health Statistics, Hyattsville, MD [online]. Available: http://www.cdc.gov/nchs/about/major/nhanes/datalink.htm [accessed June 26, 2008].

NICNAC (The National Chemicals Notification and Assessment Scheme-Australian Government). 2008. Dimethyl Phthalate. Existing Chemical Hazard Assessment

Report. Australian Government, Department of Health and Ageing, NICNAC, Sydney. June 2008 [online]. Available: http://www.nicnas.gov.au/publications/car/ other/DMP%20hazard%20asssessment.pdf [accessed Sept. 22, 2008].

Parmar, D., S.P. Srivastava, S.P. Srivastava, and P.K. Seth. 1985. Hepatic mixed function oxidases and cytochrome P-450 contents in rat pups exposed to di(2ethylhexyl)-phthalate through mother's milk. Drug Metab. Dispos. 13(3):368-370.

Pollack, G.M., J.F. Buchanan, R.L. Slaughter, R.K. Kohli, and D.D. Shen. 1985a. Circulating concentrations of di(2-ethylhexyl) phthalate and its de-esterified phthalic acid products following plasticizer exposure in patients receiving hemodialysis. Toxicol. Appl. Pharmacol. 79(2):257-267.

Pollack, G.M., R.C. Li, J.C. Ermer, and D.D. Shen. 1985b. Effects of route of administration and repetitive dosing on the disposition kinetics of di(2-ethylhexyl) phthalate and its mono-de-esterified metabolite in rats. Toxicol. Appl. Pharmacol. 79(2):246-256.

Rudel, R.A., D.E. Camann, J.D. Spengler, L.R. Korn, and J.G. Brody. 2003. Phthalates, alkylphenols, pesticides, polybrominated diphenyl ethers, and other endocrine-disrupting compounds in indoor air and dust. Environ. Sci. Technol. 37(20):4543-4553.

Saillenfait, A.M., J.P. Payan, J.P. Fabry, D. Beydon, I. Langonne, F. Gallissot, and J.P. Sabate. 1998. Assessment of the developmental toxicity, metabolism, and placental transfer of Di-n-butyl phthalate administered to pregnant rats. Toxicol. Sci. 45(2):212-224.

Sathyanarayana, S., C.J. Karr, P. Lozano, E. Brown, A.M. Calafat, F. Liu, and S.H. Swan. 2008. Baby care products: Possible sources of infant phthalate exposure. Pediatrics 121(2):e260-268.

Shea, K.M., and the AAP Committee on Environmental Health. 2003. Pediatric exposure and potential toxicity of phthalate plasticizers. Pediatrics 111(6 Pt.1):1467-1474.

Shono, T., H. Kai, S. Suita, and H. Nawata. 2000. Time-specific effects of mono-n-butyl phthalate on the transabdominal descent of the testis in rat fetuses. BJU Int. 86(1):121-125.

Silva, M.J., D.B. Barr, J.A. Reidy, K. Kato, N.A. Malek, C.C. Hodge, D. Hurtz III, A.M. Calafat, L.L. Needham, and J.W. Brock. 2003. Glucuronidation patterns of common urinary and serum monoester phthalate metabolites. Arch. Toxicol. 77(10):561-567.

Silva, M.J., J.A. Reidy, A.R. Herbert, J.L. Preau, L.L. Needham, and A.M. Calafat. 2004. Detection of phthalate metabolites in human amniotic fluid. Bull. Environ. Contam. Toxicol. 72(6):1226-1231.

Silva, M.J., E. Samandar, J.L. Preau, L.L. Needham, and A.M. Calafat. 2006. Urinary oxidative metabolites of di (2-ethylhexyl) phthalate in humans. Toxicology 219(1-3):22-32.

Silva, M.J., J.A. Reidy, K. Kato, J.L. Preau Jr., L.L. Needham, and A.M. Calafat. 2007a. Assessment of human exposure to di-isodecyl phthalate using oxidative metabolites as biomarkers. Biomarkers 12(2):133-144.

Silva, M.J., E. Samandar, J.A. Reidy, R. Hauser, L.L. Needham, and A.M. Calafat. 2007b. Metabolite profiles of di-n-butyl phthalate in humans and rats. Environ. Sci. Technol. 41(21):7576-7580.

Sjoberg, P.O., U.G. Bondesson, E.G. Sedin, and J.P. Gustafsson. 1985. Exposure of newborn infants to plasticizers. Plasma levels of di(2ethylhexyl)phthalate during exchange transfusion. Transfusion 25(5):424-428.

Sorensen, L.K. 2006. Determination of phthalates in milk and milk products by liquid chromatography/tandem mass spectrometry. Rapid. Commun. Mass Spectrom 20(7): 1135-1143.

Weuve, J., B.N. Sanchez, A.M. Calafat, T. Schettler, R.A.Green, H. Hu, and R. Hauser. 2006. Exposure to phthalates in neonatal intensive care unit infants: Urinary concentrations of monoesters and oxidative metabolites. Environ. Health Perspect. 114(9):1424-1431.

Wittassek, M., and J. Angerer. 2008. Phthalates: Metabolism and exposure. Int. J. Androl. 31(2):131-138.

Wittassek, M., G.A. Wiesmuller, H.M. Koch, R. Eckard, L. Dobler, J. Muller, J. Angerer, and C. Schluter. 2007. Internal phthalate exposure over the last two decades—a retrospective human biomonitoring study. Int. J. Hyg. Environ. Health 210(3-4):319-333.

Wolff, M.S., S.M. Engel, G.S. Berkowitz, X. Ye, M.J. Silva, C. Zhu, J. Wetmur, and A.M. Calafat. 2008. Prenatal phenol and phthalate exposures and birth outcomes. Environ. Health Perspect. 116(8):1092-1097.

3

Toxicity Assessment

The toxicity of some phthalates[1] in animals has been known for decades, although few data are available on the toxicity of these chemicals in humans. Several human studies have reported associations of exposure of some phthalates with adverse reproductive outcomes and developmental effects similar to those in the rat. However, for the purposes of this chapter, reliance will be placed on the data obtained from animal studies. Species differences (mainly quantitative) in response will be referred to in the text with citation of human data when available. As noted in Chapter 1, the outcomes chosen for emphasis in this report are effects on the development of the male reproductive system. The reproductive developmental processes in rats are analogous to those in humans, and disruption of those processes in rats should be representative of what would occur in humans if the same processes are disrupted (reviewed in Foster 2005).

This chapter first discusses male sexual differentiation in mammals. That information serves merely to provide context for the discussion that follows; references to several reviews are provided for readers who would like further information. The results of early teratology studies are mentioned, and the reproductive effects of phthalates are then discussed. Aspects of the phthalate syndrome—its relationship to the hypothesized human testicular dysgenesis syndrome, structure-activity relationships, and mechanisms of action—are described next. Agents that produce effects on reproductive development similar to those of phthalates are noted. Although cancer is not the focus of this report, carcinogenic effects were the focus of much research on phthalates in past years, so the committee felt that the chapter would not be complete without a brief discussion of them. This chapter provides the context for the discussion on cumulative risk assessment and is not meant to be a comprehensive toxicity assessment or an exhaustive review of phthalate toxicity.

---

[1]As stated in Chapter 1, the term *phthalates* used in this report refers to diesters of 1,2-benzenedicarboxylic acid, the *o*-phthalates.

MALE SEXUAL DIFFERENTIATION IN MAMMALS

Sexual differentiation in males follows complex interconnected pathways during embryo and fetal development that have been reviewed extensively elsewhere (see, for example, Capel 2000; Hughes 2001; Tilmann and Capel 2002; Brennan and Capel 2004).

Critical to the development of male mammals is the development of the testis in embryonic life from a bipotential gonad (a tissue that could develop into a testis or an ovary). The "selection" is genetically controlled in most mammals by a gene on the Y chromosome. The sex-determining gene (sry in mice and SRY in humans) acts as a switch to control multiple downstream pathways that lead to the male phenotype. Male differentiation after gonad determination is exclusively hormone-dependent and requires the presence at the correct time and tissue location of specific concentrations of fetal testis hormones—Mullerian inhibiting substance (MIS), insulin-like factors, and androgens. Although a female phenotype is produced independently of the presence of an ovary, the male phenotype depends greatly on development of the testis. Under the influence of hormones and cell products from the early testis, the Mullerian duct regresses, and the mesonephric duct (or Wolffian duct) gives rise to the epididymis and vas deferens. In the absence of MIS and testosterone, the Mullerian ductal system develops further into the oviduct, uterus, and upper vagina, and the Wolffian duct system regresses. Those early events occur before the establishment of a hypothalamic-pituitary-gonadal axis and depend on local control and production of hormones (that is, the process is gonadotropin-independent). Normal development and differentiation of the prostate from the urogenital sinus and of the external genitalia from the genital tubercle are also under androgen control. More recent studies of conditional knockout mice that have alterations of the luteinizing-hormone receptor have shown normal differentiation of the genitalia, although they are significantly smaller.

Testis descent (see Figure 3-1) appears to require androgens and the hormone insulin-like factor 3 (insl3; Adham et al. 2000) to proceed normally. The testis in early fetal life is near the kidney and attached to the abdominal wall by the cranial suspensory ligament (CSL) and gubernaculum. The gubernaculum contracts, thickens, and develops a bulbous outgrowth; this results in the location of the testis in the lower abdomen (transabdominal descent). The CSL regresses through an androgen-dependent process. In the female, the CSL is retained with a thin gubernaculum to maintain ovarian position. Descent of the testes through the inguinal ring into the scrotum (inguinoscrotal descent) is under androgen control.

Because the majority of studies discussed below were conducted in rats, it is helpful to compare the rat and human developmental periods for male sexual differentiation (see Figure 3-2). Production of fetal testosterone occurs over a broader window in humans (gestation weeks 8-37) than in rats (gestation days [GD] 15-21). The critical period for sexual differentiation in humans is late in

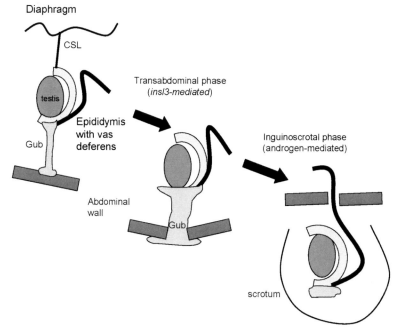

FIGURE 3-1 Stages of testicular descent. Testicular descent in scrotal mammals (such as humans and rats) can be conveniently divided into two phases. The first is the transabdominal phase in which the cranial suspensory ligament (CSL) disappears, and the testes—located near the kidneys—move into the lower abdomen. The first phase is under the control of the hormone, insulin-like factor 3. The second phase is the inguinoscrotal phase in which the gubernaculum (Gub) develops further, and the testes move through the body wall (inguinal ring) into the developing scrotum. The second phase is under the control of androgen. Source: Klonisch et al. 2004. Reprinted with permission; copyright 2004, *Developmental Biology*.

the first trimester of pregnancy, and differentiation is essentially complete by 16 weeks (Hiort and Holterhus 2000). The critical period in rats occurs in later gestation, as indicated by the production of testosterone in the latter part of the gestational period, and some sexual development occurs postnatally in rats. For example, descent of the testis into the scrotum occurs in gestation weeks 27-35 in humans and in the third postnatal week in rats. Generally, the early postnatal period in rats corresponds to the third trimester in humans.

    Given the above discussion, it is clear that normal differentiation of the male phenotype has specific requirements for fetal testicular hormones, including androgens, and therefore can be particularly sensitive to the action of environmental agents that can alter the endocrine milieu of the fetal testis during critical periods of development.

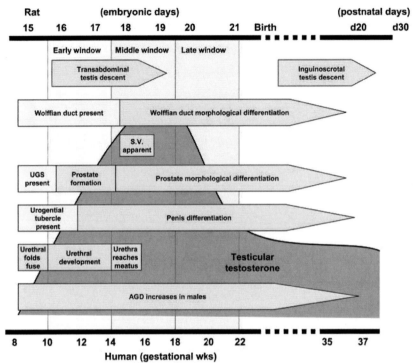

FIGURE 3-2 Comparison of periods of male reproductive development in rat and human. The shaded area under the curve indicates the changing testosterone concentrations in the fetal testis. Gestational weeks (humans) were measured from time of last menstrual period, so birth occurs at 40 weeks in this diagram. S.V., seminal vesicles. Source: Welsh et al. 2008. Reprinted with permission; copyright 2008, *Clinical Investigation.*

EARLY TERATOLOGY FINDINGS

The early studies that examined the potential for phthalate exposure to cause adverse effects on fetal development were standard teratology studies, in which pregnant animals were exposed during GD 6-15, and the offspring were examined just before birth, when the reproductive tract is immature. Generally, the concentration of a phthalate required to cause developmental toxicity in those studies was relatively high, and maternal toxicity was typically observed (NTP 2000, 2003a,b,c,d,e,f, 2006). Typical malformations observed included neural-tube defects, cleft palate, and skeletal abnormalities. On the basis of the early data, the National Toxicology Program (NTP) and its Center for the Evaluation of Risks to Human Reproduction (CERHR) (NTP 2000, 2003a,b,c,d,e,f, 2006) concluded that there was clear evidence of adverse developmental effects in animals for BBP, DBP, DEHP, and DIDP and some evidence for DINP but only limited evidence for DHP and DOP. However, as discussed further below, the design of the standard teratology study was shown to be inadequate for detecting the spectrum of male reproductive effects that have now been reported because of their failure to include exposure during critical gestational windows.

REPRODUCTIVE EFFECTS

The testis was identified as a target organ in some of the first toxicity studies undertaken with phthalates (see, for example, Gray et al. 1977). Although the effects in young adult animals were seen only at high doses in rat studies, it was obvious that testicular lesions could be produced with relatively short-term dosing models. Those lesions were the most severe manifestations of testicular toxicity in that there was complete tubular atrophy. Initial experiments also indicated that there was an age sensitivity: pubertal animals had effects at doses lower than those in the corresponding studies in adult animals.

Investigations of structure-activity relationships in the pubertal-rat model showed that the ester side-chain length of linear-chain phthalates needed to be four to six carbon atoms to produce testicular toxicity (Foster et al. 1980). Di-*n*-pentyl phthalate was the most potent in producing testicular toxicity. Phthalates of one to three carbons (methyl, ethyl, and *n*-propyl) did not produce testicular toxicity when given at a dose equimolar with DBP at 2 g/kg-d. Similarly, linear-chain phthalates of seven or eight carbons did not produce adverse effects. DEHP, which has eight carbons and a branched structure, had activity more similar to that of di-*n*-hexyl phthalate than to its linear isomer di-*n*-octyl phthalate. Investigation of the isomers of DBP indicated that the esters needed to be in the *ortho* configuration in that equimolar doses of the *n*-butyl esters in the *meta*- and *para*- positions were without effect in the pubertal-rat model (Foster et al. 1981a). Other studies with butyl phthalates indicated that the *iso* and *sec* esters were equivalent to the *n*-butyl but that the *tert* ester was without effect at equimolar doses (Foster et al. 1981b).

Detailed morphologic examination of the phthalate-induced testicular lesions in pubertal rats (Foster et al. 1982; Creasy et al. 1983) and adult rats (Creasy et al. 1987) indicated that the Sertoli cell was the initial testicular target and that loss of support of the germ cells resulted in their rapid sloughing into the seminiferous tubular lumen, which resulted in a spermatogenic stage-specific lesion in adult animals. The effects of the various *n*-alkyl phthalates could be modeled with in vitro systems of mixed Sertoli and germ cell cultures (Gray and Beamand 1984), which demonstrated the same structure-activity relationships as that described for in vivo testicular toxicity. The in vitro Sertoli cell culture systems also provided some insight into a potential mechanism of action for the pubertal model; effects on responsiveness of follicle-stimulating hormone were noted (Lloyd and Foster 1988; Heindel and Chapin 1989). Other in vitro studies of developing Sertoli cells and gonocytes taken from neonatal animals indicated that these cells showed an even greater sensitivity to phthalates than did the cells derived from pubertal animals; the increased sensitivity could be reproduced in neonatal rat pups (Li et al. 1998, 2000; Li and Kim 2003).

The number of known environmental agents that produce adverse testicular responses in male humans is not large, and although there may be differences in sensitivity based on dose, all of them have been shown to induce effects in rodents, especially the rat. Accordingly, most of the studies of effects of phthalates on male reproduction have been conducted in rodents, primarily rats. Gray et al. (1982) evaluated species differences in the induction of testicular toxicity of DBP and DEHP in the rat, mouse, guinea pig, and hamster. They found that the rat was the most sensitive, the guinea pig was broadly equivalent, the mouse was much less sensitive, and the hamster was resistant. The differences in testicular toxicity were suggested to be due largely to pharmacokinetic differences. The results for the guinea pig were in stark contrast with the species differences observed in effects on the induction of hepatic growth and peroxisome proliferation. The lower male reproductive toxicity observed for the mouse was consistent with the results of other studies of reproductive toxicants. For example, a number of the classic human testicular toxicants, such as 1,2-dibromo-3-chloropropane (Oakberg and Cummings 1984) and gossypol (Hahn et al. 1981; Kalla et al. 1990), do not seem to produce infertility or testicular toxicity in the mouse, so the rat is more commonly used as a model for male reproductive-toxicity studies. Although that does not imply that all agents known to produce injury in the rat would cause toxicity in humans, it does suggest that the rat is generally a good model of human male reproductive toxicity.

The ability of specific phthalates to alter reproductive development in utero was first demonstrated by a multigeneration study of DBP in the rat by NTP (NTP 1991; Wine et al. 1997), although the critical nature of the effects was not immediately recognized. In that study (see Table 3-1), the highest dose of DBP (1% in the diet) produced few functional effects on the parental generation; all the exposed males were able to sire litters, but decreases in litter size were noted. However, only one of 20 F_1 males produced a litter at the same 1% dietary dose, and this indicated the importance of exposure during early life (gestation and lactation and up to puberty) as a contributing factor. The number of underdeveloped epididymides in F_1 males and the presence of other rare reproductive tract malformations recorded at low incidence were also noteworthy. The adverse effects on the development of the reproductive system were not reported in the standard prenatal developmental toxicity studies. It was later discovered that the exposure period in the standard studies (from implantation to the closure of the hard palate, GD 6-15 in the rat) does not cover the critical developmental window, now known to be GD 15-17 for phthalates (Carruthers and Foster 2005; see Figure 3-3). The U.S. Environmental Protection Agency (EPA 1998) has since extended the dosing period in its guidelines for prenatal developmental toxicity testing to GD 6-20 (in the rat) to avoid some of the pitfalls inherent when agents that might affect the development of the reproductive

TABLE 3-1 Reproductive and Developmental Effects of DBP in the National Toxicology Program Reproductive Assessment by Continuous Breeding Study (1991)

Effect Noted	F_0 Generation	F_1 Generation
Decrease in fertility	–	+
Decrease in litter size (of fertile animals)	+	+
Decrease in testes weight (and histopathology)	–	+
Decrease in pup weight	+	+
Decrease in sperm count	–	+
Cryptorchidism	Not applicable	+
Male reproductive tract malformations (epididymide, external genitalia)	Not applicable	+
Female reproductive tract weight (and histopathology)	–	–
Estrus cyclicity	–	–

Note: +, positive response; –, negative response.

system are evaluated. However, there has been no change in the time of examination of fetuses (usually just before term—around GD 21 in rats), so diagnosis of reproductive tract malformations remains problematic. It was only when the DBP multigeneration study was followed up with a more defined exposure period (Mylchreest et al. 1998, 1999) that the increased sensitivity of the fetus to DBP was described (Mylchreest et al. 2000).

THE PHTHALATE SYNDROME OF EFFECTS ON MALE REPRODUCTIVE DEVELOPMENT

Since the recognition of the critical importance of exposure during GD 15-17, many studies have been conducted to determine the full spectrum of effects that can result from exposure to phthalates in utero. Studies have shown that male rats exposed to biologically active phthalates in utero during the period of sexual differentiation exhibit a number of reproductive tract abnormalities, which may include underdeveloped or absent reproductive organs, malformed external genitalia (hypospadias), undescended testes (cryptorchidism), decreased anogenital distance, retained nipples, and decreased sperm production (Mylchreest et al. 1998, 1999; Gray et al. 2000). Studies evaluating DBP found that the fetal testes of phthalate-exposed males are characterized by seminiferous cords that contain multinucleated gonocytes (Barlow and Foster 2003; Hutchison et al. 2008). Phthalate exposure also results in regions of Leydig cell hyperplasia. Barlow et al. (2004) showed that a small percentage of male offspring

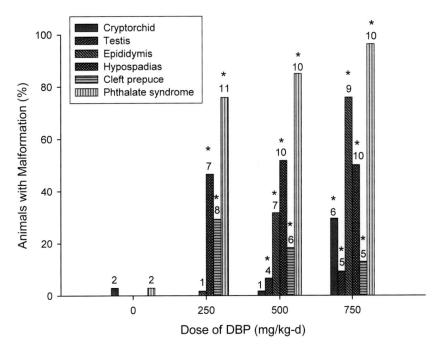

* P < 0.05 (Fisher's exact)

FIGURE 3-3 Effect of DBP given over 3 days on reproductive tract malformations. Pregnant Sprague-Dawley rats were given DBP on GD 15-17, critical window for induction of phthalate syndrome, at 0, 250, 500, or 750 mg/kg-d by gavage in corn oil (5 mL/kg-d). Reproductive tract malformations were assessed in male offspring at postnatal day 100. Litters (10-12) were evaluated in each dose group; numbers of litters responding are indicated above bars. Control animals exhibited only cryptorchidism. Only when exposure occurred over GD 15-17 was the full suite of reproductive tract malformations that make up the phthalate syndrome observed. Other short-term (2-d) dosing regimens over GD 15-20 will produce specific reproductive malformations but not the full suite of malformations (Carruthers and Foster 2005).

exposed to DBP in utero also develop Leydig cell adenomas as early as the age of 3 months. As discussed above, younger rodents are more sensitive to the adverse testicular effects of phthalates than older rodents. Pubertal and prepubertal rodents are more sensitive to the adverse effects of phthalates on the testes than adults (Foster et al. 1980; Sjoberg et al. 1986, 1988), and the fetal testes respond to phthalate concentrations that would be without effect in pubertal or adult animals (Gray et al. 2000; Mylchreest et al. 2000; Lehmann et al. 2004). Thus, the pubertal and prepubertal rat is sensitive, but the prenatal period is the most sensitive time for the testicular effects of phthalates.

Testicular Dysgenesis Syndrome

Human males exhibit a high incidence of reproductive disorders. Cryptorchidism and hypospadias are the most common male birth defects. In the United States, cryptorchidism affects 2-4% of male newborns (Barthold and Gonzalez 2003), and hypospadias occur in about one of 250 male newborns (Paulozzi et al. 1997).[2] The incidence of male germ-cell cancers is thought to be on the rise (Skakkebæk et al. 2001), and studies suggest that semen quality has been decreasing (Carlsen et al. 1992; Swan et al. 2000). Testicular germ-cell cancers arise from abnormal fetal germ cells (Rajpert-De Meyts et al. 1998; Rorth et al. 2000), and disorders of sperm production may also arise during gestation (Sharpe and Franks 2002). The above disorders are risk factors for each other and share other pregnancy-related risk factors (Skakkebæk et al. 2001). On the basis of those observations, it has been hypothesized that they comprise a "testicular dysgenesis syndrome," which arises in fetal life during reproductive system development because of disruption of critical gene programming in the fetal testis by either genetic or environmental factors (Skakkebæk et al. 2001; Sharpe and Skakkebæk 2008). The actions of phthalates on the developing reproductive tract of male rats exhibit excellent concordance with the end points of concern in the human male population that make up the testicular dysgenesis syndrome (see Table 3-2). However, there are no human data that directly link phthalate exposure with the hypothesized syndrome.

TABLE 3-2 Comparison of Human Male Reproductive Effects of Concern with Effects of in Utero Phthalate Exposure in Rats

Human Reproductive Effects with a Possible in Utero Origin	Effects of in Utero Phthalate Exposure in Rats
Infertility	√
Decreased sperm count	√
Cryptorchidism	√
Reproductive tract malformations	√
Hypospadias	√
Testicular tumors[a]	√[a]

[a]Testicular tumors in rats are Leydig-cell-derived, not germ-cell-derived as in humans.

---

[2]There is some uncertainty in the rates reported, which depend on diagnostic criteria and on the time at which evaluation is conducted. Some subtle changes are not always noted, and newborns have a different incidence of cryptorchidism from infants at 6 months. Moreover, prospective studies with defined diagnostic criteria tend to provide better information than studies using registry data.

Structure-Activity Relationships

As discussed above, high-dose acute oral exposure to various *n*-alkyl phthalates induced testicular toxicity in pubertal rats and revealed differences in activity based on chemical structure (Foster et al. 1980). The studies indicated that only phthalates with chain lengths of four to six carbon atoms were capable of inducing testicular damage; di-*n*-pentyl phthalate yielded the most severe response. DEHP had toxicity that more closely resembled that induced by *n*-hexyl phthalate rather than that induced by its isomer di-*n*-octyl phthalate, which was without testicular toxicity. That observation indicated that branching of the ester side chain was also important. A similar structure-activity relationship has been demonstrated after in utero exposure (Gray et al. 2000). Phthalates with chain lengths of four to six carbons (dibutyl, butylbenzyl, dipentyl, and diethyl-hexyl) reduced fetal testicular testosterone and impaired male reproductive development, whereas phthalates with shorter or longer side chains (dimethyl, di-ethyl, and dioctyl) did not have an effect on male reproductive development (see Table 3-3).[3] The developmentally toxic phthalates are indistinguishable in their effects on global gene expression in the fetal testis (Liu et al. 2005). The common targeting of specific fetal testis genes by a select group of phthalates indicates common molecular mechanisms of action.

Mechanism of Action

The primary target of phthalates after in utero exposure is the fetal testis. One of the earliest phthalate-related fetal effects observed in rats was disturbance of fetal testicular Leydig cell function or development (Parks et al. 2000; Shultz et al. 2001; Mylchreest et al. 2002; Fisher et al. 2003). That disturbance results in large aggregates of fetal Leydig cells (at GD 21) in the developing testis. The morphologic changes were preceded by a decrease in fetal testicular production of the androgen testosterone, which reached only 10% of control concentrations in some animals (Shultz et al. 2001; Lehmann et al. 2004; Howdeshell et al. 2008). Androgen insufficiency at critical times in male reproductive system development results in the failure of the Wolffian duct system to develop normally into the vas deferens, epididymis, and seminal vesicles (Barlow and Foster 2003). Lower testosterone concentrations also affect the dihydro-testosterone (DHT)-induced development of the prostate and external genitalia (testosterone is converted to DHT by 5α-reductase). DHT is also responsible for the normal apoptosis of nipple anlagen[4] in males, which results in the lack of

---

[3]Although DIBP is strictly considered a phthalate with a chain length of three carbons, it produced toxicity similar to that of DBP.

[4]Anlagen is defined as a precursor tissue.

TABLE 3-3 Effect of in Utero Phthalate Exposure on Male Rat Reproductive Outcomes

Phthalate	Phthalate Syndrome	Doses (mg/kg-d)	Lowest Observed-Effect Level (mg/kg-d)	Effect Observed	Reference
DMP	–	750		–	Gray et al. 2000
DEP	–	750		–	Gray et al. 2000
DBP	+	0.1, 1.0, 10, 30, 50, 100, 500	50	Reduced testosterone	Lehmann et al. 2004
DIBP	+	100, 300, 600, 900	300	Reduced testosterone	Howdeshell et al. 2008
BBP	+	50, 250, 750	250	Reduced anogenital distance	Tyl et al. 2004
Di-*n*-pentyl	+	25, 50, 100, 200, 300, 600, 900	100	Reduced testosterone	Howdeshell et al. 2008
DEHP	+	0.09-0.12, 0.47-0.78, 1.4-2.4, 4.8-7.9, 14-23, 46-77, 392-592, 543-775	14-23	Reduced reproductive organ weight	NTP 2004
DCHP	+	18, 90, 457	90	Reduced anogenital distance	Hoshino et al. 2005
DINP	+	750	750	Nipple retention	Gray et al. 2000

nipple development, and for the growth of the perineum to produce the normal male anogenital distance (AGD), about twice that of the female (Imperato-McGinley et al. 1985, 1986). Thus, the observed changes in androgen-dependent developmental landmarks are consistent with the lowered fetal concentrations of testosterone.

Separately from effects on testosterone synthesis, in utero phthalate exposure disrupts seminiferous cord formation and germ-cell development and leads to the appearance of large multinucleated germ cells in late gestation (Mylchreest et al. 2002; Barlow and Foster 2003; Kleymenova et al. 2005). The multinucleated germ cells disappear postnatally. Germ-cell maturation is delayed in phthalate-exposed fetal testes. Postnatally, there is a delay in the resumption of germ-cell mitosis, and germ-cell number and presumably sperm count are reduced (Sharpe 2008).

As discussed above (see Figure 3-1), testicular descent into the scrotum requires normal androgen concentrations and insl3 (Adham et al. 2000), and a failure of descent results in cryptorchidism (George 1989; Imperato-McGinley et al. 1992). After DEHP, DBP, or BBP exposure in utero, a decrease in expression of insl3 gene was noted in rat fetal testes (Lehmann et al. 2004; Wilson et al. 2004). The decrease may be related to the increased incidence of cryptorchidism after fetal exposure to phthalates. Knockouts of the insl3 gene in mice show complete cryptorchidism (Nef and Parada 1999; Nef et al. 2000). Although human polymorphisms of insl3 have not been reported, polymorphisms of the insl3 receptor (LGR8), which has recently been shown to be related to cryptorchidism in humans, have been noted (Ivell and Hartung 2003).

The Phthalate Syndrome in Other Species

Although the actions of phthalates on male reproductive development have been studied primarily in the rat, aspects of the phthalate syndrome have also been demonstrated in other species. Adverse testicular effects have been noted in rabbits (Higuchi et al. 2003) and ferrets (Lake et al. 1976). A recent study of the effect of in utero exposure to phthalates in the mouse showed that phthalates do not suppress testosterone synthesis or insl3 production in the fetal testis. Despite an overall lack of an effect on testicular testosterone steroidogenesis, DBP exposure impaired seminiferous cord formation and induced gonocyte multinucleation in the mouse (Gaido et al. 2007). As discussed above, the rat is generally considered a more relevant model than the mouse for the study of reproductive and developmental toxicity.

Most studies of nonhuman primates have failed to show effects on adult testicular function (reviewed in Matsumoto et al. 2008); this finding is not surprising, given that adult rats are also much less sensitive than their fetal or pubertal counterparts. There has, however, been one report of effects on developing testicular Leydig cells and decreased testosterone concentrations in the neonatal marmoset (Hallmark et al. 2007) that are similar to the changes in rats, although concerns have been raised about the relevance of the marmoset model (Li et al. 2005).

There have been reports of an association between phthalate exposure and reduction in semen quality in humans (Duty et al. 2003; Hauser et al. 2006). Like the animal studies, the human studies found associations between urinary concentrations of MBP and reduced semen quality. However, the human studies did not find associations between MEHP and reduced semen quality, and this is inconsistent with the animal data.

A few small studies of humans have linked maternal exposure to specific phthalate metabolites, found in either urine or breast milk, with adverse outcomes in the children, including shortened AGD (Swan et al. 2005; Marsee et al. 2006; Swan 2006) and decreased free testosterone concentrations in infant boys (Main et al. 2006). The associations are similar to the findings noted above in rats with, for example, DBP (AGD is one of the most sensitive rat end points). However, the associations reported in human and animal studies are not always analogous. For example, positive correlations between DEP exposure and effects have been noted in human studies, but DEP exposure does not cause the phthalate syndrome in animals. The positive findings on DEP in humans on which animal data have been negative, may reflect its coexposure with other phthalates (see Chapter 2), differences between rodent and human toxicity, or other biologic factors. The results obtained thus far are intriguing, but additional research is needed to confirm them.

Effects of Phthalate Exposure in Females

Effects of phthalates on female reproductive function have received far less attention than effects in the male primarily because of the high doses required to induce functional effects. A series of studies probed the effects of various phthalates on ovarian granulosa-cell function, particularly steroid production (Davis et al. 1994a,b; Lovekamp and Davis 2001; Lovekamp-Swan and Davis 2003) in the ovary that led to anovulation at high doses of DEHP. A recent study (Gray et al. 2006), however, indicated that long-term exposure to DBP at 500 mg/kg-d may result in a failure of the pregnant dam to maintain pregnancy because of a decrease in ovarian progesterone production; that dose is far below the DEHP dosage of 2 g/kg-d required to induce anovulation. Few adverse effects on the female reproductive system have been reported in nonrodents. A few human case studies are available but have not been replicated, such as one that noted the relationship of phthalate exposure to the presence of endometriosis (Reddy et al. 2006).

AGENTS THAT PRODUCE SIMILAR EFFECTS ON REPRODUCTIVE DEVELOPMENT

Although the spectrum of effects of some phthalates on male reproductive development in utero in rats is specific (the phthalate syndrome), a number of other types of agents can produce similar outcomes through a perturbation in androgen concentrations or androgen-receptor (AR) signaling. Indeed, in many of the reproductive tissues that require androgen for their normal development, it is unlikely that one can differentiate between a decreased concentration of the ligand (testosterone or DHT) and a blockade of the AR; the response or consequences would be identical, producing common adverse outcomes (see Figure 3-4).

Although inhibition of insl3 appears unique to the effects of phthalates, some phthalates can reduce fetal testicular testosterone production. That property is shared by an array of agents that can produce "androgen insufficiency" in the developing fetus, which in turn can yield effects on male reproductive devel-

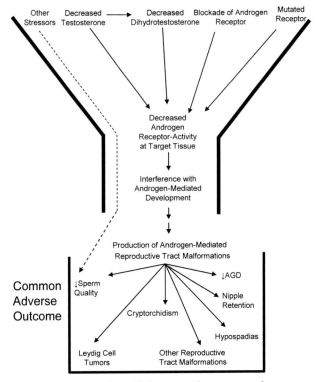

FIGURE 3-4 Fetal androgen insufficiency and common adverse outcomes.

opment that would include many of the same malformations caused by phthalates. The processes that would be affected would include the development of the Wolffian duct into the epididymis, vas deferens, and seminal vesicle (predominantly under the control of testosterone) and the development of the urogenital sinus into the prostate and the genital tubercle, which develops into the penis (all of which are predominantly under DHT control). Effects on the length of the perineum (AGD) and apoptosis of the nipple anlagen in rats are also under DHT control. Indeed, the syndrome of androgen insufficiency could be considered a subset of the phthalate syndrome, with only the effects on insl3 and germ-cell development being different. Figure 3-5 shows the relationship between the phthalate syndrome and the androgen-insufficiency effects and compares the phthalate syndrome noted in rats with the hypothesized human testicular dysgenesis syndrome. There is a remarkable overlap in response between the phthalate syndrome and the hypothesized human testicular dysgenesis syndrome, except for responses for which rats are sexually dimorphic (retention of nipples) or that rodents do not exhibit (for example, rats do not develop

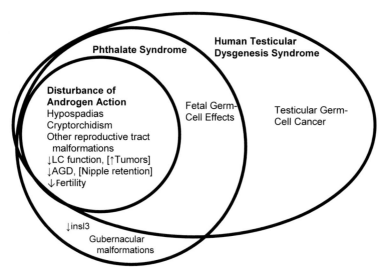

FIGURE 3-5 Relationship of phthalate syndrome in rats to that noted for agents that perturb androgen action to produce androgen insufficiency and to the hypothesized testicular dysgenesis syndrome in humans. End points in brackets are restricted to findings in experimental animals.

testicular germ-cell cancer—the most common cancer in young men—but rather Leydig cell tumors of the testis, which are commonly noted both spontaneously and after exposure to biologically active phthalates). However, there are no human data that directly link the hypothesized human syndrome with phthalate exposure.

The agents that can produce androgen insufficiency can be loosely grouped into three main classes: AR antagonist, mixed-function inhibitors, and 5α-reductase inhibitors. The spectrum of induced malformations is similar to that of phthalates, but the precise tissue sensitivity and therefore the most common malformations observed after in utero exposure to each group are different.

Androgen-Receptor Antagonists

AR antagonists constitute the true pharmacologic antiandrogens and cover a broad array of structures from pharmaceuticals, such as flutamide, to agricultural fungicides, such as vinclozolin and procymidone. They can bind competitively to the AR and can produce a suite of malformations, particularly at low doses on tissues under DHT control, including some of the changes in AGD and nipple retention noted for phthalates. The most common malformations observed in rats after administration of flutamide are prostatic malformations and hypospadias (see, for example, McIntyre et al. 2001), and similar changes are noted after exposure to vinclozolin (Gray et al. 1999a; Gray et al. 1993) or procymidone (Gray et al. 1999b; Ostby et al. 1999). *p,p'*-Dichlorodiphenyl di-chloroethylene (*p,p'*-DDE), the major metabolite of the insecticide DDT, was the first environmental antiandrogen reported (Kelce et al. 1995), although it has activity in vivo as an AR antagonist (Kelce et al. 1997), the phenotype observed is typically weaker than that of the other AR antagonists mentioned above.

Mixed-Function Inhibitors

A number of environmental agents have been shown to have multiple mo-lecular mechanisms by which they induce androgen insufficiency after exposure of rats in utero. Collectively, the agents can both reduce fetal testicular testoster-one production (as phthalates can) and be AR antagonists. The tissue selectivity will depend on the relative potency for each of those activities. Although the herbicide linuron is a competitive AR antagonist (McIntyre et al. 2000), the pre-dominant malformation is of the epididymis (McIntyre et al. 2000, 2002a,b; Turner et al. 2003)—a phenotype much more similar to that noted after fetal testicular testosterone inhibition by phthalates (the epididymis being the site of the most prevalent malformation). Hotchkiss et al. (2004) showed that linuron could indeed reduce fetal testicular testosterone production. In contrast, the fun-gicide prochloraz produces effects on male reproductive development and is an AR antagonist (Noriega et al. 2005; Vinggaard et al. 2005), but the predominant malformations that it causes more closely resemble those seen with vinclozolin (in the production of hypospadias) than those associated with phthalates. Pro-chloraz does inhibit CYP 17 to produce a reduction in fetal testicular testoster-one (Blystone et al. 2007) and also antagonizes aromatase (CYP 19) activity (Sanderson et al. 2002; Vinggaard et al. 2005).

5α-Reductase Inhibitors

A number of drugs can specifically inhibit the conversion of testosterone to DHT. If administration occurs in utero in rats, such inhibition leads to the production of specific malformations of the male reproductive tract that would require DHT for their normal development. They tend to involve tissues more remote from the testes and more typical of the malformations noted with AR antagonists. Finasteride is a classic example of a drug in this class; when admin-istered in utero to dams during the period of male sexual differentiation, it can produce a wide array of male reproductive tract malformations (see, for exam-ple, Bowman et al. 2003), the most predominant being hypospadias. Not surpris-ingly, permanent reductions in AGD and retention of nipples (processes that normally require DHT to establish the male phenotype) were noted at even lower doses than those that produced malformations. Because testosterone con-centrations were unaltered, none of the typical epididymal effects of phthalates and of some mixed-function inhibitors was observed with this 5α-reductase in-hibitor.

Comparison of Agents

Table 3-4 indicates the variety of predominant malformations associated with the different molecular mechanisms. The overall spectrum of induced malformations resulting from disturbances in androgen concentration is very similar to that resulting from disturbances in signaling. Although there might be quantitative differences in the individual malformations produced, depending on precise mechanisms or doses, the similarity in response of the androgen-dependent organs indicates that few independent pathways of response exist in relation to androgen disturbances. Thus, a developing prostate seems to respond in the same manner irrespective of the agent that lowers the concentration of a ligand, whether testosterone or DHT, or that blocks or alters signaling of the AR in the target tissue. Accordingly, the prostatic malformations induced by phthalates (which lower fetal testicular testosterone production), AR antagonists (such as flutamide and vinclozolin), mixed acting agents (such as prochloraz), and the 5α-reductase inhibitor finasteride are identical.

TABLE 3-4 Effects of Agents That Can Produce Androgen Insufficiency by Different Pharmacologic Activities or Mechanisms and the Most Common Resulting Malformation after in Utero Exposure of Pregnant Rats during Sexual Differentiation

Agent	↓Androgen-Receptor Activity	↓Insl3 Activity	↓Testosterone or Dihydrotestosterone Concentrations	Most Commonly Observed Malformations
Vinclozolin, Procymidone, Flutamide	+	–	–	Hypospadias
Linuron	+	–	+	Epididymal and testicular abnormalities No gubernacular agenesis
Prochloraz	+	–	+	Hypospadias
Finasteride	–	–	+	Hypospadias
DBP, DIBP, BBP, DPP, DEHP, DIHP, DINP, DCHP	–	+	+	Epididymal and testicular abnormalities Gubernacular agenesis
DEP, DMP	–	–	–	No malformations noted

+, known pharmacologic activity; –, no activity.

CANCER

This chapter has primarily addressed male reproductive effects of phthalates. However, much research on phthalate toxicity has focused on the carcinogenic effects observed in animal models. One of the best described carcinogenic effects of phthalates is hepatic cancer, although hepatic neoplasms are not observed in response to long-term exposure of all phthalates. Evidence from multiple reports (reviewed in NTP 2000) demonstrates that DEHP and DINP cause hepatic tumors in rats and mice (Table 3-5). Some phthalate monoesters—including MEHP, MINP, MBP, MBZP, MOP, and MIDP—can activate peroxisome-proliferator-activated receptor-α (PPARα), as demonstrated by Bility et al. (2004), who used an in vitro reporter assay. The ability of phthalate monoesters to activate PPARα increases with increasing chain length. Generally, the mouse PPARα can be activated by lower concentrations of the phthalate monoesters than can the human PPARα, and the response of the mouse PPARα is much greater than that of the human PPARα (Bility et al. 2004). Accordingly, DEHP and DINP are thought to cause hepatocarcinogenesis through their monoester metabolites at relatively high exposure because of ligand activation of PPARα, which is known to mediate hepatocarcinogenic effects in rodents (Peters et al. 1997; Hays et al. 2005).

TABLE 3-5 Summary of Hepatocarcinogenic Effects of Phthalates

Species	Sex	NOEL (mg/kg-d)	LOEL (mg/kg-d)	Reference
DINP				
Rat	Male	359	700	Lington et al. 1997
Mouse	Male	275	742	Moore 1998
Mouse	Female	112	336	Moore 1998
DEHP				
Rat	Male	95	300	Voss et al. 2005
Mouse	Male	674	–	Kluwe 1986
Mouse	Female	394	774	Kluwe 1986
Rat	Male	–	672	Kluwe 1986
Rat	Female	–	799	Kluwe 1986
Mouse	Male	19	99	David et al. 1999
Mouse	Female	117	354	David et al. 1999
Rat	Male	29	147	David et al. 1999
Rat	Female	183	939	David et al. 1999

NOTE: LOEL, lowest observed-effect level; NOEL, no-observed-effect level.

A recent study in mice, however, suggests that DEHP-induced hepatocarcinogenesis occurs in the absence of PPARα expression. Ito et al. (2007) exposed wild-type and PPARα-null-type mice to 0.01% and 0.05% DEHP in the diet. The wild-type mice showed no statistically significant differences in hepatocarcinogenesis. However, a significant trend for an increase in total hepatic tumors was observed at 0.05% DEHP in PPARα-null-type mice compared with control PPARα-null-type mice. Although PPARα-null-type mice exhibit a high background incidence of hepatocarcinogenesis (Howroyd et al. 2004), statistical comparisons were made within the same groups; therefore, that fact should not have affected the reported results. Thus, the results suggest that DEHP might cause hepatic cancer in rodents through a mechanism that is independent of PPARα, as has been suggested by others (see, for example, Takashima et al. 2008).

There is a known difference between rodents and humans in the ability of PPARα ligands to cause changes in the liver, including increases in cell growth and peroxisome proliferation (Peters et al. 2005), and it has been suggested that the hepatocarcinogenic effects of DEHP and DINP are unlikely to occur in humans (Klaunig et al. 2003). More recent evidence supports that idea: mice that express human PPARα in the absence of mouse PPARα are refractory to the hepatocarcinogenic effects of PPARα ligands (Morimura et al. 2006). The lack of a hepatocarcinogenic effect of PPARα ligands in the "humanized" mouse model appears to be due to a species-specific differential regulation of a microRNA that regulates c-myc, an oncogene that is thought to be involved in cell proliferation (Shah et al. 2007). The differential regulation of this microRNA might also explain the lack of changes in hepatic markers of cell proliferation observed in nonhuman primates exposed to DEHP or DINP (Rhodes et al. 1986; Pugh et al. 2000). However, whether exposure to PPARα ligands, such as phthalates, causes hepatic cancer in humans is unclear; further research is needed to answer this question definitively (Peters et al. 2005).

In addition to hepatic cancer, some phthalates can cause tumors in other cell types. For example, a "tumor triad"—liver tumors, testicular Leydig cell tumors, and pancreatic acinar-cell tumors—has been described for some PPARα ligands, such as DEHP (Klaunig et al. 2003). BBP causes hepatic cancer and pancreatic acinar-cell tumors but not Leydig cell tumors (NTP 1997). It has been postulated that pancreatic acinar-cell tumors and Leydig cell tumors may also be mediated by PPARα (Klaunig et al. 2003). There are known species differences in response to PPARα ligands in the liver that appear to be mediated by differential changes in gene expression that lead to differences in c-myc expression, and similar differences in PPARα-mediated events suggest that humans might not be susceptible to the nonhepatic tumors. However, further work is necessary to establish those putative PPARα-dependent mechanisms in the testicular Leydig cell tumors and the pancreatic acinar-cell tumors because the current evidence supporting those mechanisms is not strong (Klaunig et al. 2003). Thus, the nonhepatic tumors reported to occur after phthalate exposure in animal models may be mediated through mechanisms that are independent of PPARα.

CONCLUSIONS

In undertaking an examination of agents that produce a syndrome of developmental response, such as the phthalate syndrome, it is normal to observe an increase in the appearance, severity, or frequency of the different malformations as the dose administered to the pregnant animal or fetus increases. Not all the animals would exhibit the full suite of malformations even at high doses, and at low doses only some of the specific effects may be manifested. It is the change in severity and frequency with respect to dose that is used to include specific agents in the characterization of specific developmental syndromes, such as the two syndromes described here (the phthalate and androgen-insufficiency syndromes). Other agents may, for example, interfere with AR action by the sequestration of cofactors after binding to other nuclear receptors, such as the aryl hydrocarbon receptor (AhR). However, none of the AhR ligands has been shown to elicit the full suite of adverse outcomes that have been described in connection with more classical antiandrogens, and such agents have therefore not been included in the committee's description of androgen insufficiency (see also Chapter 5).

As noted previously and illustrated in Figure 3-5, the phthalate syndrome observed in rats has parallels with the hypothesized human testicular dysgenesis syndrome (Sharpe 2001; Fisher et al. 2003; Joensen et al. 2008; Schumacher et al. 2008; Sharpe and Skakkebæk 2008) and shows similarities to other known human genetic syndromes involving impaired androgen responsiveness in the sexual differentiation of the reproductive tract (for a review, see Hughes 2001). Humans, in common with all mammals, have a specific requirement for androgen for the normal differentiation of the male reproductive tract during fetal life. Androgen insufficiency is well described in humans with a focus on 5α-reductase deficiencies or alteration in AR structure and function (see reviews Brinkmann 2001; Sultan et al. 2002), and disorders of androgen action are the main cause of male pseudohermaphroditism and can result in a wide spectrum of under virilization in male offspring ranging from complete external feminization to male infertility. Thus, the pathways for the critical action of androgens during fetal life are highly conserved and operate in humans as they do in experimental animals. It is biologically plausible that adverse reproductive outcomes could occur if specific phthalates or mixtures of phthalates reach the developing human fetus at the appropriate concentration and in the appropriate developmental window.

REFERENCES

Adham, I.M., J.M. Emmen, and W. Engel. 2000. The role of the testicular factor INSL3 in establishing the gonadal position. Mol. Cell Endocrinol. 160(1-2):11-16.
Barlow, N.J., and P.M. Foster. 2003. Pathogenesis of male reproductive tract lesions from gestation through adulthood following in utero exposure to di(*n*-butyl) phthalate. Toxicol. Pathol. 31(4): 397-410.

Barlow, N.J., B.S. McIntyre, and P.M. Foster. 2004. Male reproductive tract lesions at 6, 12, and 18 months of age following in utero exposure to di(*n*-butyl) phthalate. Toxicol. Pathol. 32(1):79-90.

Barthold, J.S., and R. Gonzalez. 2003. The epidemiology of congenital cryptorchidism, testicular ascent and orchiopexy. J. Urol. 170(6 Pt 1):2396-2401.

Bility, M.T., J.T. Thompson, R.H. McKee, R.M. David, J.H. Butala, J.P. Vanden Heuvel, and J.M. Peters. 2004. Activation of mouse and human peroxisome proliferator-activated receptors (PPARs) by phthalate monoesters. Toxicol. Sci. 82(1):170-182.

Blystone, C.R., C.S. Lambright, K.L. Howdeshell, J. Furr, R.M. Sternberg, B.C. Butterworth, E.J. Durhan, E.A. Makynen, G.T. Ankley, V.S. Wilson, G.A. Leblanc, and L.E. Gray, Jr. 2007. Sensitivity of fetal rat testicular steroidogenesis to maternal prochloraz exposure and the underlying mechanism of inhibition. Toxicol. Sci. 97(2):512-519.

Bowman, C.J., N.J. Barlow, K.J. Turner, D.G. Wallace, and P.M. Foster. 2003. Effects of in utero exposure to finasteride on androgen-dependent reproductive development in the male rat. Toxicol. Sci. 74(2):393-406.

Brennan, J., and B. Capel. 2004. One tissue, two fates: Molecular genetic events that underlie testis versus ovary development. Nat. Rev. Genet. 5(7):509-521.

Brinkmann, A.O. 2001. Molecular basis of androgen insensitivity. Mol. Cell Endocrinol. 179(1-2):105-109.

Capel, B. 2000. The battle of the sexes. Mech. Dev. 92(1):89-103.

Carlsen, E., A. Giwercman, N. Keiding, and N.E. Skakkebæk. 1992. Evidence for decreasing quality of semen during past 50 years. BMJ 305(6854):609-613.

Carruthers, C.M., and P.M. Foster. 2005. Critical window of male reproductive tract development in rats following gestational exposure to di-*n*-butyl phthalate. Birth Defects Res. B Dev. Reprod. Toxicol. 74(3):277-285.

Creasy, D.M., J.R. Foster, and P.M. Foster. 1983. The morphological development of di-n-pentyl phthalate induced testicular atrophy in the rat. J. Pathol. 139(3):309-321.

Creasy, D.M., L.M. Beech, T.J. Gray, and W.H. Butler. 1987. The ultrastructural effects of di-n-pentyl phthalate on the testis of the mature rat. Exp. Mol. Pathol. 46(3):357-371.

David, R.M., M.R. Moore, M.A. Cifone, D.C. Finney, and D. Guest. 1999. Chronic peroxisome proliferation and hepatomegaly associated with the hepatocellular tumorigenesis of di(2-ethylhexyl)phthalate and the effects of recovery. Toxicol. Sci. 50(2):195-205.

Davis, B.J., R.R. Maronpot, and J.J. Heindel. 1994a. Di-(2-ethylhexyl) phthalate suppresses estradiol and ovulation in cycling rats. Toxicol. Appl. Pharmacol. 128(2):216-223.

Davis, B.J., R. Weaver, L.J. Gaines, and J.J. Heindel. 1994b. Mono-(2-ethylhexyl) phthalate suppresses estradiol production independent of FSH-cAMP stimulation in rat granulosa cells. Toxicol. Appl. Pharmacol. 128(2):224-228.

Duty, S.M., M.J. Silva, D.B. Barr, J.W. Brock, L. Ryan, Z. Chen, R.F. Herrick, D.C. Christiani, and R. Hauser. 2003. Phthalate exposure and human semen parameters. Epidemiology 14(3):269-277.

EPA (U.S. Environmental Protection Agency). 1998. Health Effects Test Guidelines OPPTS 870.3700 Prenatal Developmental Toxicity Study. EPA712-C-98-207. Office of Prevention, Pesticides and Toxic Substances, U.S. Environmental Protection Agency, Washington, DC. August 1998 [online]. Available: http://www.epa.gov/opptsfrs/publications/OPPTS_Harmonized/870_Health_Effects_Test_Guidelines/Series/870-3700.pdf [accessed Sept. 24, 2008].

Fisher, J.S., S. Macpherson, N. Marchetti, and R.M. Sharpe. 2003. Human testicular dysgenesis syndrome: A possible model using in-utero exposure of the rat to dibutyl
phthalate. Hum. Reprod. 18(7):1383-1394.

Foster, P.M. 2005. Mode of action: Impaired fetal Leydig cell function-effects on male
reproductive development produced by certain phthalate esters. Crit. Rev. Toxicol.
35(8-9):713-719.

Foster, P.M., L.V. Thomas, M.W. Cook, and S.D. Gangolli. 1980. Study of the testicular
effects and changes in zinc excretion produced by some n-alkyl phthalates in the
rat. Toxicol. Appl. Pharmacol. 54(3):392-398.

Foster, P.M., B.G. Lake, M.W. Cook, L.V. Thomas, and S.D. Gangolli. 1981a. Structure-activity requirements for the induction of testicular atrophy by butyl phthalates in immature rats: Effect on testicular zinc content. Adv. Exp. Med. Biol. 136
Pt A:445-452.

Foster, P.M., B.G. Lake, L.V. Thomas, M.W. Cook, and S.D. Gangolli. 1981b. Studies
on the testicular effects and zinc excretion produced by various isomers of mono-
butyl-o-phthalate in the rat. Chem. Biol. Interact. 34(2):233-238.

Foster, P.M., J.R. Foster, M.W. Cook, L.V. Thomas, and S.D. Gangolli. 1982. Changes in
ultrastructure and cytochemical localization of zinc in rat testis following the administration of di-n-pentyl phthalate. Toxicol. Appl. Pharmacol. 63(1):120-132.

Gaido, K.W., J.B. Hensley, D. Liu, D.G. Wallace, S. Borghoff, K.J. Johnson, S.J. Hall,
and K. Boekelheide. 2007. Fetal mouse phthalate exposure shows that Gonocyte
multinucleation is not associated with decreased testicular testosterone. Toxicol.
Sci. 97(2):491-503.

George, F.W. 1989. Developmental pattern of 5 alpha-reductase activity in the rat gubernaculum. Endocrinology 124(2):727-732.

Gray, L.E., J.M. Ostby, and R. Marshall. 1993. The fungicide vinclozolin inhibits morphological sex differentiation in the male rat. Biol. Reprod. 48 (Suppl. 1):97.

Gray, L.E., Jr., J. Ostby, E. Monosson, and W.R. Kelce. 1999a. Environmental antiandrogens: Low doses of the fungicide vinclozolin alter sexual differentiation of the
male rat. Toxicol. Ind. Health 15(1-2):48-64.

Gray, L.E., Jr., C. Wolf, C. Lambright, P. Mann, M. Price, R.L. Cooper, and J. Ostby.
1999b. Administration of potentially antiandrogenic pesticides (procymidone, linuron, iprodione, chlozolinate, p,p'-DDE, and ketoconazole) and toxic substances
(dibutyl- and diethylhexyl phthalate, PCB 169, and ethane dimethane sulphonate)
during sexual differentiation produces diverse profiles of reproductive malformations in the male rat. Toxicol. Ind. Health 15(1-2):94-118.

Gray, L.E., Jr., J. Ostby, J. Furr, M. Price, D.N. Veeramachaneni, and L. Parks. 2000.
Perinatal exposure to the phthalates DEHP, BBP, and DINP, but not DEP, DMP,
or DOTP, alters sexual differentiation of the male rat. Toxicol. Sci. 58(2):350-365.

Gray, L.E., Jr., J. Laskey, and J. Ostby. 2006. Chronic di-n-butyl phthalate exposure in
rats reduces fertility and alters ovarian function during pregnancy in female Long
Evans hooded rats. Toxicol. Sci. 93(1):189-195.

Gray, T.J., and J.A. Beamand. 1984. Effect of some phthalate esters and other testicular
toxins on primary cultures of testicular cells. Food Chem. Toxicol. 22(2):123-131.

Gray, T.J., K.R. Butterworth, I.F. Gaunt, G.P. Grasso, and S.D. Gangolli. 1977. Short-
term toxicity study of di-(2-ethylhexyl) phthalate in rats. Food Cosmet. Toxicol.
15(5):389-399.

Gray, T.J., I.R. Rowland, P.M. Foster, and S.D. Gangolli. 1982. Species differences in
the testicular toxicity of phthalate esters. Toxicol. Lett. 11(1-2):141-147.

Hahn, D.W., C. Rusticus, A. Probst, R. Homm, and A.N. Johnson. 1981. Antifertility and endocrine activities of gossypol in rodents. Contraception 24(1):97-105.

Hallmark, N., M. Walker, C. McKinnell, I.K. Mahood, H. Scott, R. Bayne, S. Coutts, R.A. Anderson, I. Greig, K. Morris, and R.M. Sharpe. 2007. Effects of monobutyl and di(*n*-butyl) phthalate in vitro on steroidogenesis and Leydig cell aggregation in fetal testis explants from the rat: Comparison with effects in vivo in the fetal rat and neonatal marmoset and in vitro in the human. Environ. Health Perspect. 115(3):390-396.

Hauser, R., J.D. Meeker, S. Duty, M.J. Silva, and A.M. Calafat. 2006. Altered semen quality in relation to urinary concentrations of phthalate monoester and oxidative metabolites. Epidemiology 17(6): 682-691.

Hays, T., I. Rusyn, A.M. Burns, M.J. Kennett, J.M. Ward, F.J. Gonzalez, and J.M. Peters. 2005. Role of peroxisome proliferator-activated receptor-{alpha} (PPARalpha) in bezafibrate-induced hepatocarcinogenesis and cholestasis. Carcinogenesis 26(1):219-227.

Heindel, J.J., and R.E. Chapin. 1989. Inhibition of FSH-stimulated cyclic AMP accumulation by mono-(2-ethylhexyl) phthalate in primary rat Sertoli cell cultures. Toxicol. Appl. Pharmacol. 97(2): 377-385.

Higuchi, T.T., J.S. Palmer, L.E. Gray, Jr., and D.N. Veeramachaneni. 2003. Effects of dibutyl phthalate in male rabbits following in utero, adolescent, or postpubertal exposure. Toxicol. Sci. 72(2):301-313.

Hiort, O., and P.M. Holterhus. 2000. The molecular basis of male sexual differentiation. Eur. J. Endocrinol. 142(2):101-110.

Hoshino, N., M. Iwai, and Y. Okazaki. 2005. A two-generation reproductive toxicity study of dicyclohexyl phthalate in rats. J. Toxicol. Sci. 30(Spec. No.):79-96.

Hotchkiss, A.K., L.G. Parks-Saldutti, J.S. Ostby, C. Lambright, J. Furr, J.G. Vandenbergh, and L.E. Gray, Jr. 2004. A mixture of the "antiandrogens" linuron and butyl benzyl phthalate alters sexual differentiation of the male rat in a cumulative fashion. Biol. Reprod. 71(6):1852-1861.

Howdeshell, K.L., V.S. Wilson, J. Furr, C.R. Lambright, C.V. Rider, C.R. Blystone, A.K. Hotchkiss, and L.E. Gray, Jr. 2008. A mixture of five phthalate esters inhibits fetal testicular testosterone production in the Sprague-Dawley rat in a cumulative, dose-additive manner. Toxicol. Sci. 105(1):153-165.

Howroyd, P., C. Swanson, C. Dunn, R.C. Cattley, and J.C. Corton. 2004. Decreased longevity and enhancement of age-dependent lesions in mice lacking the nuclear receptor peroxisome proliferator-activated receptor alpha (PPARalpha). Toxicol. Pathol. 32(5):591-599.

Hughes, I.A. 2001. Minireview: Sex differentiation. Endocrinology 142(8):3281-3287.

Hutchison, G.R., R.M. Sharpe, I.K. Mahood, M. Jobling, M. Walker, C. McKinnell, J.I. Mason, and H.M. Scott. 2008. The origins and time of appearance of focal testicular dysgenesis in an animal model of testicular dysgenesis syndrome: Evidence for delayed testis development? Int. J. Androl. 31(2): 103-111.

Imperato-McGinley, J., Z. Binienda, A. Arthur, D.T. Mininberg, E.D. Vaughan, Jr., and F.W. Quimby. 1985. The development of a male pseudohermaphroditic rat using an inhibitor of the enzyme 5 alpha-reductase. Endocrinology 116(2):807-812.

Imperato-McGinley, J., Z. Binienda, J. Gedney, and E.D. Vaughan, Jr. 1986. Nipple differentiation in fetal male rats treated with an inhibitor of the enzyme 5 alpha-reductase: Definition of a selective role for dihydrotestosterone. Endocrinology 118(1):132-137.

Imperato-McGinley, J., R.S. Sanchez, J.R. Spencer, B. Yee, and E.D. Vaughan. 1992. Comparison of the effects of the 5 alpha-reductase inhibitor finasteride and the antiandrogen flutamide on prostate and genital differentiation: Dose-response studies. Endocrinology 131(3):1149-1156.

Ito, Y., O. Yamanoshita, N. Asaeda, Y. Tagawa, C.H. Lee, T. Aoyama, G. Ichihara, K. Furuhashi, M. Kamijima, F.J. Gonzalez, and T. Nakajima. 2007. Di(2-ethylhexyl)-phthalate induces hepatic tumorigenesis through a peroxisome proliferator-activated receptor alpha-independent pathway. J. Occup. Health 49(3):172-182.

Ivell, R., and S. Hartung. 2003. The molecular basis of cryptorchidism. Mol. Hum. Reprod. 9(4):175-181.

Joensen, U.N., N. Jorgensen, E. Rajpert-De Meyts, and N.E. Skakkebæk. 2008. Testicular dysgenesis syndrome and Leydig cell function. Basic Clin. Pharmacol. Toxicol. 102(2):155-161.

Kalla, N.R., A. Ranga, R.K. Vyas, N. Gadru, and J. Foo. 1990. Response of mice testis to gossypol acetic acid. Acta Eur. Fertil. 21(1):17-19.

Kelce, W.R., C.R. Stone, S.C. Laws, L.E. Gray, J.A. Kemppainen, and E.M. Wilson. 1995. Persistent DDT metabolite p,p'-DDE is a potent androgen receptor antagonist. Nature 375(6532):581-585.

Kelce, W.R., C.R. Lambright, L.E. Gray, Jr., and K.P. Roberts. 1997. Vinclozlin and *p,p'*-DDE alter androgen-dependent gene expression: In vivo confirmation of an androgen receptor-mediated mechanism. Toxicol. Appl. Pharmacol. 142(1):192-200.

Klaunig, J.E., M.A. Babich, K.P. Baetcke, J.C. Cook, J.C. Corton, R.M. David, J.G. DeLuca, D.Y. Lai, R.H. McKee, J.M. Peters, R.A. Roberts, and P.A. Fenner-Crisp. 2003. PPARalpha agonist-induced rodent tumors: Modes of action and human relevance. Crit. Rev. Toxicol. 33(6):655-780.

Kleymenova, E., C. Swanson, K. Boekelheide, and K.W. Gaido. 2005. Exposure in utero to di(*n*-butyl) phthalate alters the vimentin cytoskeleton of fetal rat Sertoli cells and disrupts Sertoli cell-gonocyte contact. Biol. Reprod. 73(3):482-490.

Klonisch, T., P.A. Fowler, and S. Hombach-Klonisch. 2004. Molecular and genetic regulation of testis descent and external genitalia development. Dev. Biol. 270(1):1-18.

Kluwe, W.M. 1986. Carcinogenic potential of phthalic acid esters and related compounds: Structure-activity relationships. Environ. Health Perspect. 65:271-278.

Lake, B.G., P.G. Brantom, S.D. Gangolli, K.R. Butterworth, and P. Grasso. 1976. Studies on the effects of orally administered Di-(2-ethylhexyl) phthalate in the ferret. Toxicology 6(3):341-356.

Lehmann, K.P., S. Phillips, M. Sar, P.M. Foster, and K.W. Gaido. 2004. Dose-dependent alterations in gene expression and testosterone synthesis in the fetal testes of male rats exposed to di (n-butyl) phthalate. Toxicol. Sci. 81(1):60-68.

Li, H., and K.H. Kim. 2003. Effects of mono-(2-ethylhexyl) phthalate on fetal and neonatal rat testis organ cultures. Biol. Reprod. 69(6):1964-1972.

Li, L.H., W.F. Jester, Jr., and J.M. Orth. 1998. Effects of relatively low levels of mono-(2-ethylhexyl) phthalate on cocultured Sertoli cells and gonocytes from neonatal rats. Toxicol. Appl. Pharmacol. 153(2):258-265.

Li, L.H., W.F. Jester, Jr., A.L. Laslett, and J.M. Orth. 2000. A single dose of di-(2-ethylhexyl) phthalate in neonatal rats alters gonocytes, reduces sertoli cell proliferation, and decreases cyclin D2 expression. Toxicol. Appl. Pharmacol. 166(3):222-229.

Li, L.H., J.M. Donald, and M.S. Golub. 2005. Review on testicular development, structure, function, and regulation in common marmoset. Birth Defects Res. B Dev. Reprod. Toxicol. 74(5):450-469.

Lington, A.W., M.G. Bird, R.T. Plutnick, W.A. Stubblefield, and R.A. Scala. 1997. Chronic toxicity and carcinogenic evaluation of diisononyl phthalate in rats. Fundam. Appl. Toxicol. 36(1):79-89.

Liu, K., K.P. Lehmann, M. Sar, S.S. Young, and K.W. Gaido. 2005. Gene expression profiling following in utero exposure to phthalate esters reveals new gene targets in the etiology of testicular dysgenesis. Biol. Reprod. 73(1):180-192.

Lloyd, S.C., and P.M. Foster. 1988. Effect of mono-(2-ethylhexyl)phthalate on follicle-stimulating hormone responsiveness of cultured rat Sertoli cells. Toxicol. Appl. Pharmacol. 95(3):484-489.

Lovekamp, T.N., and B.J. Davis. 2001. Mono-(2-ethylhexyl) phthalate suppresses aromatase transcript levels and estradiol production in cultured rat granulosa cells. Toxicol. Appl. Pharmacol. 172(3): 217-224.

Lovekamp-Swan, T., and B.J. Davis. 2003. Mechanisms of phthalate ester toxicity in the female reproductive system. Environ. Health Perspect. 111(2):139-146.

Main, K.M., G.K. Mortensen, M.M. Kaleva, K.A. Boisen, I.N. Damgaard, M. Chellakooty, I.M. Schmidt, A.M. Suomi, H.E. Virtanen, D.V. Petersen, A.M. Andersson, J. Toppari, and N.E. Skakkebæk. 2006. Human breast milk contamination with phthalates and alterations of endogenous reproductive hormones in infants three months of age. Environ. Health Perspect. 114(2):270-276.

Marsee, K., T.J. Woodruff, D.A. Axelrad, A.M. Calafat, and S.H. Swan. 2006. Estimated daily phthalate exposures in a population of mothers of male infants exhibiting reduced anogenital distance. Environ. Health Perspect. 114(6):805-809.

Matsumoto, M., M. Hirata-Koizumi, and M. Ema. 2008. Potential adverse effects of phthalic acid esters on human health: A review of recent studies on reproduction. Regul. Toxicol. Pharmacol. 50(1):37-49.

McIntyre, B.S., N.J. Barlow, D.G. Wallace, S.C. Maness, K.W. Gaido, and P.M. Foster. 2000. Effects of in utero exposure to linuron on androgen-dependent reproductive development in the male Crl:CD(SD)BR rat. Toxicol. Appl. Pharmacol. 167(2):87-99.

McIntyre, B.S., N.J. Barlow, and P.M. Foster. 2001. Androgen-mediated development in male rat offspring exposed to flutamide in utero: Permanence and correlation of early postnatal changes in anogenital distance and nipple retention with malformations in androgen-dependent tissues. Toxicol. Sci. 62(2):236-249.

McIntyre, B.S., N.J. Barlow, and P.M. Foster. 2002a. Male rats exposed to linuron in utero exhibit permanent changes in anogenital distance, nipple retention, and epididymal malformations that result in subsequent testicular atrophy. Toxicol. Sci. 65(1):62-70.

McIntyre, B.S., N.J. Barlow, M. Sar, D.G. Wallace, and P.M. Foster. 2002b. Effects of in utero linuron exposure on rat Wolffian duct development. Reprod. Toxicol. 16(2):131-139.

Moore, M.R. 1998. Oncogenicity Study in Mice with Di(isononyl)phthalate Including Ancillary Hepatocellular Proliferation and Biochemical Analyses, Vol. 1. Covance 2598-105. Covance Laboratories Incorporated, Vienna, VA. January 29, 1998.

Morimura, K., C. Cheung, J.M. Ward, J.K. Reddy, and F.J. Gonzalez. 2006. Differential susceptibility of mice humanized for peroxisome proliferator-activated receptor α to Wy-14,643-induced liver tumorigenesis. Carcinogenesis 27(5):1074-1080.

Mylchreest, E., R.C. Cattley, and P.M. Foster. 1998. Male reproductive tract malformations in rats following gestational and lactational exposure to di(*n*-butyl) phthalate: An antiandrogenic mechanism? Toxicol. Sci. 43(1):47-60.

Mylchreest, E., M. Sar, R.C. Cattley, and P.M. Foster. 1999. Disruption of androgen-regulated male reproductive development by di(*n*-butyl) phthalate during late gestation in rats is different from flutamide. Toxicol. Appl. Pharmacol. 156(2):81-95.

Mylchreest, E., D.G. Wallace, R.C. Cattley, and P.M. Foster. 2000. Dose-dependent alterations in androgen-regulated male reproductive development in rats exposed to di(*n*-butyl) phthalate during late gestation. Toxicol. Sci. 55(1):143-151.

Mylchreest, E., M. Sar, D.G. Wallace, and P.M. Foster. 2002. Fetal testosterone insufficiency and abnormal proliferation of Leydig cells and gonocytes in rats exposed to di(*n*-butyl) phthalate. Reprod. Toxicol. 16(1):19-28.

Nef, S., and L.F. Parada. 1999. Cryptorchidism in mice mutant for Insl3. Nat. Genet. 22(3):295-299.

Nef, S., T. Shipman, and L.F. Parada. 2000. A molecular basis for estrogen-induced cryptorchidism. Dev. Biol. 224(2):354-361.

Noriega, N.C., J. Ostby, C. Lambright, V.S. Wilson, and L.E. Gray, Jr. 2005. Late gestational exposure to the fungicide prochloraz delays the onset of parturition and causes reproductive malformations in male but not female rat offspring. Biol. Reprod. 72(6):1324-1335.

NTP (National Toxicology Program). 1991. Final Report on the Reproductive Toxicity of Di-N-Butyl Phthalate (CAS. No. 84-74-2) in Sprague-Dawley Rats. T-0035C. NTIS PB92-111996. U.S. Department of Health and Human Services, Public Health Service, National Institute of Health, National Toxicology Program, Research Triangle Park, NC.

NTP (National Toxicology Program). 1997. Effect of Dietary Restriction on Toxicology and Carcinogenesis Studies in F344/N Rats and B6C3F1 Mice. Technical Report 460. NIH 97-3376. U.S. Department of Health and Human Services, Public Health Service, National Institute of Health, National Toxicology Program, Research Triangle Park, NC.

NTP (National Toxicology Program). 2000. NTP-CERHR Expert Panel Report on Di(2-ethylhexyl) phthalate. NTP-CERHR-00. U.S. Department of Health and Human Services, National Toxicology Program, Center for the Evaluation of Risks to Human Reproduction. October 2000 [online]. Available: http://cerhr.niehs.nih.gov/chemicals/dehp/DEHP-final.pdf [accessed July 18, 2008].

NTP (National Toxicology Program). 2003a. NTP-CERHR Monograph on the Potential Human Reproductive and Developmental Effects of Butyl Benzyl Phthalate (BBP). NIH Pub. 03-4487. U.S. Department of Health and Human Services, National Toxicology Program, Center for the Evaluation of Risks to Human Reproduction. March 2003 [online]. Available: http://cerhr.niehs.nih.gov/chemicals/phthalates/bb-phthalate/BBP_Monograph_Final.pdf [accessed July 18, 2008].

NTP (National Toxicology Program). 2003b. NTP-CERHR Monograph on the Potential Human Reproductive and Developmental Effects of Di-Isodecyl Phthalate (DIDP). NIH Pub. 03-4485. U.S. Department of Health and Human Services, National Toxicology Program, Center for the Evaluation of Risks to Human Reproduction. April 2003 [online]. Available: http://cerhr.niehs.nih.gov/chemicals/phthalates/didp/DIDP_Monograph_Final.pdf [accessed July 18, 2008].

NTP (National Toxicology Program). 2003c. NTP-CERHR Monograph on the Potential Human Reproductive and Developmental Effects of Di-isononyl Phthalate (DINP). NIH Pub. 03-4484. U.S. Department of Health and Human Services, National Toxicology Program, Center for the Evaluation of Risks to Human Reproduction. March 2003 [online]. Available: http://cerhr.niehs.nih.gov/chemicals/phthalates/dinp/DiNP_Monograph_Final.pdf [accessed July 18, 2008].

NTP (National Toxicology Program). 2003d. NTP-CERHR Monograph on the Potential Human Reproductive and Developmental Effects of Di-n-Butyl Phthalate (DBP). NIH Pub. 03-4486. U.S. Department of Health and Human Services, National Toxicology Program, Center for the Evaluation of Risks to Human Reproduction. [online]. Available: http://cerhr.niehs.nih.gov/chemicals/phthalates/dbp/DBP_ Monograph_Final.pdf [accessed July 18, 2008].

NTP (National Toxicology Program). 2003e. NTP-CERHR Monograph on the Potential Human Reproductive and Developmental Effects of Di-n-Hexyl Phthalate (DnHP). NIH Pub. 03-4489 . U.S. Department of Health and Human Services, National Toxicology Program, Center for the Evaluation of Risks to Human Reproduction. May 2003 [online]. Available: http://cerhr.niehs.nih.gov/chemicals/phthalates/ dnhp/DnHP_Monograph_Final.pdf [accessed July 18, 2008].

NTP (National Toxicology Program). 2003f. NTP-CERHR Monograph on the Potential Human Reproductive and Developmental Effects of Di-n-Octyl Phthalate (DnOP). NIH Pub. 03-4488 . U.S. Department of Health and Human Services, National Toxicology Program, Center for the Evaluation of Risks to Human Reproduction. May 2003 [online]. Available: http://cerhr.niehs.nih.gov/chemicals/phthalates/ dnop/DnOP_Monograph_Final.pdf [accessed July 2008].

NTP (National Toxicology Program). 2004. Diethylhexylphthalate: Multigenerational Reproductive Assessment by Continuous Breeding When Administered to Sprague-Dawley Rats in the Diet. U.S. Department of Health and Human Services, Public Health Service, National Institute of Health, National Toxicology Program, Research Triangle Park, NC

NTP (National Toxicology Program). 2006. NTP-CERHR Monograph on the Potential Human Reproductive and Developmental Effects of Di-(2-ethylhexyl) Phthalate (DEHP). NIH Pub. 06-4476 . U.S. Department of Health and Human Services, National Toxicology Program, Center for the Evaluation of Risks to Human Reproduction. November 2006 [online]. Available: http://cerhr.niehs.nih.gov/chemicals/ dehp/DEHP-Monograph.pdf [accessed July 18, 2008].

Oakberg, E.F., and C.C. Cummings. 1984. Lack of effect of dibromochloropropane on the mouse testis. Environ. Mutagen. 6(4):621-625.

Ostby, J., W.R. Kelce, C. Lambright, C.J. Wolf, P. Mann, P., and L.E. Gray, Jr. 1999. The fungicide procymidone alters sexual differentiation in the male rat by acting as an androgen-receptor antagonist in vivo and in vitro. Toxicol. Ind. Health 15(1-2):80-93.

Parks, L.G., J.S. Ostby, C.R. Lambright, B.D. Abbott, G.R. Klinefelter, N.J. Barlow, and L.E. Gray, Jr. 2000. The plasticizer diethylhexyl phthalate induces malformations by decreasing fetal testosterone synthesis during sexual differentiation in the male rat. Toxicol. Sci. 58(2):339-349.

Paulozzi, L.J., J.D. Erickson, and R.J. Jackson. 1997. Hypospadias trends in two U.S. surveillance systems. Pediatrics 100(5):831-834.

Peters, J.M., R.C. Cattley, and F.J. Gonzalez. 1997. Role of PPAR alpha in the mechanism of action of the nongenotoxic carcinogen and peroxisome proliferator Wy-14,643. Carcinogenesis 18(11): 2029-2033.

Peters, J.M., C. Cheung, and F.J. Gonzalez. 2005. Peroxisome proliferator-activated receptor-alpha and liver cancer: Where do we stand? J. Mol. Med. 83(10):774-785.

Pugh, G., Jr., J.S. Isenberg, L.M. Kamendulis, D.C. Ackley, L.J. Clare, R. Brown, A.W. Lington, J.H. Smith, and J.E. Klaunig. 2000. Effects of di-isononyl phthalate, di-2-ethylhexyl phthalate, and clofibrate in cynomolgus monkeys. Toxicol. Sci. 56(1):181-188.

Rajpert-De Meyts, E., N. Jorgensen, K. Brondum-Nielsen, J. Muller, and N.E. Skakkebæk. 1998. Developmental arrest of germ cells in the pathogenesis of germ cell neoplasia. Acta Path. Micro. Im. C 106(1):198-206.

Reddy, B.S., R. Rozati, B.V. Reddy, and N.V. Raman. 2006. Association of phthalate esters with endometriosis in Indian women. Bjog 113(5):515-520.

Rhodes, C., T.C. Orton, I.S. Pratt, P.L. Batten, H. Bratt, S.J. Jackson, and C.R. Elcombe. 1986. Comparative pharmacokinetics and subacute toxicity of di(2-ethylhexyl) phthalate (DEHP) in rats and marmosets: Extrapolation of effects in rodents to man. Environ. Health Perspect. 65:299-307.

Rorth, M., E. Rajpert-De Meyts, L. Andersson, K.P. Dieckmann, S.D. Fossa, K.M. Grigor, W.F. Hendry, H.W. Herr, L.H. Looijenga, J.W. Oosterhuis, and N.E. Skakkebæk. 2000. Carcinoma in situ in the testis. Scand. J. Urol. Nephrol. Suppl. (205): 166-186.

Sanderson, J.T., J. Boerma, G.W. Lansbergen, and M. van den Berg. 2002. Induction and inhibition of aromatase (CYP19) activity by various classes of pesticides in H295R human adrenocortical carcinoma cells. Toxicol. Appl. Pharmacol. 182(1):44-54.

Schumacher, V., B. Gueler, L.H. Looijenga, J.U. Becker, K. Amann, R. Engers, J. Dotsch, H. Stoop, W. Schulz, and B. Royer-Pokora. 2008. Characteristics of testicular dysgenesis syndrome and decreased expression of SRY and SOX9 in Frasier syndrome. Mol. Reprod. Dev. 75(9):1484-1494.

Shah, Y.M., K. Morimura, Q. Yang, T. Tanabe, M. Takagi, and F.J. Gonzalez. 2007. Peroxisome proliferator-activated receptor alpha regulates a microRNA-mediated signaling cascade responsible for hepatocellular proliferation. Mol. Cell. Biol. 27(12):4238-4247.

Sharpe, R.M. 2001. Hormones and testis development and the possible adverse effects of environmental chemicals. Toxicol. Lett. 120(1-3):221-232.

Sharpe, R.M. 2008. An Animal Model for "Testicular Dysgenesis Syndrome" Based on in Utero Exposure to Dibutyl Phthalate (DBP): Effects of DBP on Germ Cells in the Fetal Testis. Presentation at the 2nd Meeting on Health Risks of Phthalates, February 21, 2008, Washington, DC.

Sharpe, R.M., and S. Franks. 2002. Environment, lifestyle and infertility--an intergenerational issue. Nat. Cell Biol. (Suppl. 4):s33-s40.

Sharpe, R.M., and N.E. Skakkebæk. 2008. Testicular dysgenesis syndrome: Mechanistic insights and potential new downstream effects. Fertil. Steril. 89(Suppl. 2):e33-e38.

Shultz, V.D., S. Phillips, M. Sar, P.M. Foster, and K.W. Gaido. 2001. Altered gene profiles in fetal rat testes after in utero exposure to di(n-butyl) phthalate. Toxicol. Sci. 64(2):233-242.

Sjoberg, P., N.G. Lindqvist, and L. Ploen. 1986. Age-dependent response of the rat testes to di(2-ethylhexyl) phthalate. Environ. Health Perspect. 65:237-242.

Sjoberg, P., U. Bondesson, and J. Gustafsson. 1988. Metabolism of mono-(2-ethylhexyl) phthalate in fetal, neonatal and adult rat liver. Biol. Neonate 53(1):32-38.

Skakkebæk, N.E., E. Rajpert-De Meyts, and K.M. Main. 2001. Testicular dysgenesis syndrome: An increasingly common developmental disorder with environmental aspects. Hum. Reprod. 16(5):972-978.

Sultan, C., S. Lumbroso, F. Paris, C. Jeandel, B. Terouanne, C. Belon, F. Audran, N. Poujol, V. Georget, J. Gobinet, S. Jalaguier, G. Auzou, and J.C. Nicolas. 2002. Disorders of androgen action. Semin. Reprod. Med. 20(3):217-228.

Swan, S.H. 2006. Prenatal phthalate exposure and anogenital distance in male infants. Environ. Health Perspect. 114:A88-A89.

Swan, S.H., E.P. Elkin, and L. Fenster. 2000. The question of declining sperm density revisited: An analysis of 101 studies published 1934-1996. Environ. Health Perspect. 108(10):961-966.

Swan, S.H., K.M. Main, F. Liu, S.L. Stewart, R.L. Kruse, A.M. Calafat, C.S. Mao, J.B. Redmon, C.L. Ternand, S. Sullivan, and J.L. Teague. 2005. Decrease in anogenital distance among male infants with prenatal phthalate exposure. Environ. Health Perspect. 113(8):1056-1061.

Takashima, K., Y. Ito, F.J. Gonzalez, and T. Nakajima. 2008. Different mechanisms of DEHP-induced hepatocellular adenoma tumorigenesis in wild-type and Ppar- alpha-null mice. J. Occup. Health 50(2):169-180.

Tilmann, C., and B. Capel. 2002. Cellular and molecular pathways regulating mammalian sex determination. Recent Prog. Horm. Res. 57:1-18.

Turner, K.J., B.S. McIntyre, S.L. Phillips, N.J. Barlow, C.J. Bowman, and P.M. Foster. 2003. Altered gene expression during rat Wolffian duct development in response to in utero exposure to the antiandrogen linuron. Toxicol. Sci. 74(1):114-128.

Tyl, R.W., C.B. Myers, M.C. Marr, P.A. Fail, J.C. Seely, D.R. Brine, R.A. Barter, and J.H. Butala. 2004. Reproductive toxicity evaluation of dietary butyl benzyl phthalate (BBP) in rats. Reprod. Toxicol. 18(2):241-264.

Vinggaard, A.M., S. Christiansen, P. Laier, M.E. Poulsen, V. Breinholt, K. Jarfelt, H. Jacobsen, M. Dalgaard, C. Nellemann, and U. Hass. 2005. Perinatal exposure to the fungicide prochloraz feminizes the male rat offspring. Toxicol. Sci. 85(2):886-897.

Voss, C., H. Zerban, P. Bannasch, and M.R. Berger. 2005. Lifelong exposure to di-(2-ethylhexyl)-phthalate induces tumors in liver and testes of Sprague-Dawley rats. Toxicology 206(3):359-371.

Welsh, M., P.T.K. Saunders, M. Fisken, H.M. Scott, G.R. Hutchison, L.B. Smith, and R.M. Sharpe. 2008. Identification in rats of a programming window for reproductive tract masculinization, disruption of which leads to hypospadias and cryptorchidism. Clin. Invest. 118(4):1479-1490.

Wilson, V.S., C. Lambright, J. Furr, J. Ostby, C. Wood, G. Held, and L.E. Gray. 2004. Phthalate ester-induced gubernacular lesions are associated with reduced insl3 gene expression in the fetal rat testis. Toxicol. Lett. 146(3):207-215.

Wine, R.N., L.H. Li, L.H. Barnes, D.K. Gulati, and R.E. Chapin. 1997. Reproductive toxicity of di-n-butylphthalate in a continuous breeding protocol in Sprague-Dawley rats. Environ. Health Perspect. 105(1):102-107.

4

Current Practice in Risk Assessment and Cumulative Risk Assessment

Chapter 2 summarizes the evidence on human exposure to phthalates and demonstrates that there is ample evidence of simultaneous exposure of most of or all the U.S. population to multiple phthalates. Chapter 3 examines the toxicity, as seen primarily in laboratory animal models, of individual phthalates and of other agents that produce effects similar to those seen on exposure to individual phthalates. The exposure and toxicity information clearly indicates that some sort of cumulative risk assessment is required in examining phthalate exposure. To place the discussions of Chapter 5 in context, it is useful to observe what is currently done when risks posed by multiple chemical exposures are evaluated with standard techniques according to guidance of the U.S. Environmental Protection Agency (EPA) and to examine how the guidance has evolved.

CURRENT RISK-ASSESSMENT APPROACHES AND PRACTICES

The most extensive and detailed guidance on typical risk assessments is in the *Risk Assessment Guidance for Superfund* (RAGS), particularly *Volume I, Human Health Evaluation Manual (Part A)* (EPA 1989a) and later published guidance supporting RAGS. This chapter features a description of how risk assessment is performed with RAGS because it (as intended according to its statement of purpose) tends to inform risk-assessment practice in other EPA programs and under other regulatory authorities. Additional guidance documents are cited where needed. EPA guidance on cumulative exposure and risk has evolved over the last couple of decades, and the relevant developments are discussed near the conclusion of this chapter in the section "The Evolution of Guidance on Cumulative Risk Assessment." The chapter concludes with a summary of recent cumulative exposure and risk evaluations.

The reason for considering RAGS and the actual procedures that are used in the field is to emphasize that what is done in site-specific risk assessments (for example, at Superfund sites) is distinct from the approaches and procedures used in setting standards or guidelines for individual chemicals. Although both draw heavily on toxicity assessments—for example, as appear on or are used by EPA's Integrated Risk Information System (IRIS) web site—the application of the toxicity assessments typically differs considerably between the two. Site-specific risk assessments are often concerned with simultaneous evaluation of multiple chemicals, multiple pathways of exposure, multiple routes of exposure, and multiple receptors. Standard-setting or guideline-setting generally evaluates at one time single chemicals, single routes of exposure, and single receptors, although there are exceptions, such as disinfection byproducts in drinking water.

The committee's task of evaluating the potential for a cumulative risk assessment of phthalates has to take into account that such cumulative assessments are commonly performed already, and any recommendations of the committee should be compared with the current EPA approach as described in RAGS and related guidance. Accordingly, the following sections discuss what is typically required in the exposure-assessment, toxicity-assessment, and risk-characterization parts of a risk assessment. The approaches are evaluated for what they imply about cumulative assessment of phthalates in various EPA programs, such as those involving Superfund, air toxics, and drinking water.

Exposure Assessment

The exposure-assessment component of a risk assessment of hazardous chemicals according to RAGS (EPA 1989a) requires evaluation of exposure of all the relevant, although not personally identified, people ("receptors") to all the relevant chemicals through all the relevant pathways by all the relevant routes of exposure for all relevant periods. The products of exposure assessment are estimates of exposure of defined receptors to each chemical disaggregated by periods and exposure pathways. This section provides an idealized general description, not a critical review, of the current practice of exposure assessment.

Persons Whose Exposure Is Quantified

The relevant receptors to evaluate are typically intended to be persons who experience the "reasonable maximum exposure" (RME) and persons who experience "central-tendency" (CT) exposures. The RME is the highest exposure that is expected to occur (EPA 1989a, 1992), and EPA (2001) advises that risk managers using probabilistic risk assessment should select the RME from the upper end of the range of risk estimates, "generally between the 90th and 99.9th percentiles" (EPA 2001). Later discussion focuses on persons who experience the RME because their exposure usually forms the basis of EPA decision-making (CT estimates may be needed for some pathways of the RME, as described below).

Chemicals Warranting Quantitative Dose Estimation

The relevant chemicals to evaluate in an exposure assessment are those which pass an initial screening evaluation that is used to eliminate chemicals that are clearly of no concern. The evaluation will typically first examine any available observations for frequency of occurrence and concentrations of chemicals in whatever physical media have been examined; this eliminates chemicals that occur very rarely and at concentrations much lower than risk-based screening values—precalculated values that, if they were carried through a risk assessment, would result in risk estimates small enough to be ignored. Where the only concern is increments of exposure above background, chemicals whose concentrations are similar to background may also be eliminated from further consideration. Further screening may be performed to demonstrate that even worst-case exposures (based on upper-bound estimates of exposure) present no hazard.

An exposure assessment is typically applied for many chemicals, although usually the nature of the expected major contamination is known to some degree. For example, the initial list of chemicals to be evaluated in a typical site risk assessment is usually the Contract Laboratory Program Target Compound and Target Analyte List (TCP/TAL, see EPA 2008a), combined with any site-specific chemicals known to be present and to have potential toxicity. The TCP/TAL (as of May 2008) includes 52 volatile chemicals, 30 pesticides and Aroclors, 23 metals, cyanide, and 67 semivolatile chemicals. The semivolatile chemicals include six phthalates: DMP, DEP, DBP, BBP, DEHP, and DOP.

For an exposure assessment performed for a risk assessment at a contaminated site—for example, a Superfund site or a site evaluated under similar state programs—environmental samples will often be tested for all chemicals on the TCP/TAL or similar lists, augmented where necessary. An initial screening for the full list of chemicals may be performed on a small number of samples chosen from areas thought to be most contaminated (for example, because of visual observation of soil staining, according to known locations of potentially contaminating processes, or on the basis of on-site screening with vapor detectors or conductivity measurements), and chemicals that are not detected may be dropped from the analytic sample suite. Later samples may be analyzed for a smaller list of chemicals. As discussed above, not all the chemicals analyzed will be evaluated through all parts of the exposure and risk assessment; application of screening approaches may allow chemicals to be dropped from some exposure pathways or for some receptors. For some sites or situations, there will be evaluation of special compounds not included in the lists described or special analyses of the compounds listed. For example, where contamination by poly-chlorinated dibenzo-*p*-dioxins (PCDDs) or polychlorinated dibenzo-*p*-furans (PCDFs) is suspected or found in an initial screening, analyses of various PCDD or PCDF congeners may be conducted.

Exposure Pathways and Periods Evaluated

Exposure assessment should take account of all the exposure pathways that can occur for any person. The relevant pathways included are all those by which some chemical may travel and cause exposure to the chosen receptors (that is, complete pathways). The relevant routes of exposure (ingestion, inhalation, and dermal contact) are all that may occur at the end of any particular pathway; in special circumstances, other routes, such as injection or transmucosal absorption, might have to be considered. The relevant periods depend on the toxic characteristics of the chemicals evaluated and on the timing and pattern of exposure but typically are handled by estimating exposure averaged over fixed periods for various locations and characteristics of receptors—such as age, susceptibility, and habits. Typically, assessments will evaluate acute exposure (from instantaneous to a few days long), subchronic exposure (from a few days to about 7 years), and chronic exposure (extending to a lifetime).

Total Doses Estimated for Each Receptor

For each pathway, the exposures of the receptor who experiences the RME are obtained by using procedures that result in estimates at the upper end of likely exposures, but the extent of any underestimation or overestimation is not generally known. More complex procedures, such as probabilistic methods, may be used to obtain better estimates of explicit percentiles of the exposure distribution. If it is determined that combined exposure (from multiple pathways) can occur, receptors who experience the RME are defined for combinations, and upper-end estimates of combined exposures are obtained by summing suitable combinations of estimates for each pathway. Such combinations may involve upper-end estimates for one or more pathways and average estimates for others. The aim is to obtain exposure estimates that are at the upper end of the actual or potential exposure. The result is a total dose estimate for each receptor, disaggregated by chemical, route of exposure, and period.

Toxicity Assessment

As in the preceding section, this section provides an idealized general description, not a critical review, of the current practice of toxicity assessment.

General Approach

The practical and most commonly adopted approach to toxicity assessment in EPA risk assessments is to obtain toxicity values from the EPA IRIS database for chronic oral reference doses (RfDs), chronic inhalation reference concentrations (RfCs), cancer classification, ingestion and inhalation cancer slope factors (CSFs for lifetime exposure), and inhalation and ingestion unit risks (URs for lifetime exposure). (See Box 4-1 for how those quantities are defined by EPA on its IRIS web site.[1]) In some cases, such as that of vinyl chloride, IRIS provides modifications of the values, for example, separate estimates of oral CSF or UR for continuous lifetime exposure during adulthood and for continuous lifetime exposure from birth.

BOX 4-1 EPA Definitions for Toxicity Values

Cancer Evaluations

Cancer slope factor (CSF): An upper bound, approximating a 95% confidence limit, on the increased cancer risk from a lifetime exposure to an agent. This estimate, usually expressed in units of proportion (of a population) affected per mg/kg-day, is generally reserved for use in the low-dose region of the dose-response relationship, that is, for exposures corresponding to risks less than 1 in 100.

Unit risk (UR): The upper-bound excess lifetime cancer risk estimated to result from continuous exposure to an agent at a concentration of 1 µg/L in water, or 1 µg/m^3 in air. The interpretation of unit risk would be as follows: if unit risk = 2 x 10^{-6} per µg/L, 2 excess cancer cases (upper bound estimate) are expected to develop per 1,000,000 people if exposed daily for a lifetime to 1 µg of the chemical in 1 liter of drinking water.

Noncancer Evaluations

Reference concentration (RfC): An estimate (with uncertainty spanning perhaps an order of magnitude) of a continuous inhalation exposure to the human population (including sensitive subgroups) that is likely to be without an appreciable risk of deleterious effects during a lifetime. It can be derived from a NOAEL [no-observed-adverse-effect level], LOAEL [lowest observed-adverse-effect level], or benchmark concentration, with uncertainty factors generally applied to reflect limitations of the data used.

Reference dose (RfD): An estimate (with uncertainty spanning perhaps an order of magnitude) of a daily oral exposure to the human population (including sensitive subgroups) that is likely to be without an appreciable risk of deleterious effects during a lifetime. It can be derived from a NOAEL, LOAEL, or benchmark dose, with uncertainty factors generally applied to reflect limitations of the data used.

Source: EPA 2008b.

---

[1]The committee has not examined whether the values used by EPA meet the definitions.

IRIS is at the top of EPA's recommended three-tier hierarchy of sources for toxicity values for use at Superfund sites (EPA 1993a, 2003a); more broadly, IRIS values support EPA policy-making activities (EPA 2008c). When IRIS does not provide toxicity values or when toxicity values are needed for circumstances not typically provided for in IRIS (for example, for evaluation of subchronic or acute exposures[2]), the recommended hierarchy of sources is searched sequentially for suitable values. However, EPA recognizes that the hierarchy does not address situations where new toxicity information is brought to its attention. Therefore, although in practice risk assessments typically incorporate previously developed toxicity values, especially IRIS values, new information could result in the development and application of toxicity values other than those in EPA's hierarchy.

The derivation of toxicity values for non-EPA risk assessments, such as those performed for or by state agencies, typically follows the same patterns as for EPA's risk assessments for Superfund sites. Toxicity values are typically predefined by a state agency with jurisdiction, usually by reference to a hierarchy of sources of toxicity values prepared by other suitably authoritative sources, although the hierarchy may differ from EPA's and from state to state.

The Environmental Protection Agency's IRIS Process

The output of the IRIS process is a set of toxicity values that can be used in site-specific risk assessment, such as for Superfund sites; product-specific risk assessments, such as those for consumer products; media-specific risk assessments, such as for drinking-water standards; and other applications of risk assessment. Those conducting the risk assessments must confirm the relevance of IRIS values for the chemical species, exposure pathway, exposure timeframe (nearly all toxicity values on IRIS apply to the evaluation of chronic exposures), and population under evaluation (for example, in case the population might have increased susceptibility with respect to life stage, disease status, or genetic predisposition that is not already accounted for in development of the toxicity value). The IRIS database on a chemical contains the toxicity values and brief summaries of toxicity data and other information that support them. Since 1997, the database summaries have been supplemented by detailed toxicologic reviews that undergo an independent expert peer review, including the opportunity for public review and comment. Toxicologic reviews summarize a chemical's properties, toxicokinetics, pharmacokinetic modeling where available, hazard identification based on epidemiologic studies, animal studies, in vivo and in vitro assays, and mechanism-of-action and dose-response data and culminate in quantitative recommendations for toxicity values when sufficient data are

---

[2]A recent exceptional case that provides values for subchronic and acute exposures is that of 1,1,1-trichloroethane (see EPA 2007a).

available to support them. In conducting toxicologic reviews, EPA uses relevant guidance that includes evaluation of the array of possible health outcomes, such as cancer, neurotoxicity, developmental toxicity, and reproductive toxicity.

Toxicity Values Currently Available for Phthalates

Table 4-1 summarizes toxicity values currently available for phthalates in the EPA hierarchy of sources.[3] IRIS provides a limited set of toxicity values for five phthalates. As discussed earlier, IRIS values make up the highest tier in EPA's hierarchy of toxicity values (EPA 2003a), and EPA generally favors their use, when available, over lower-tier toxicity values. Provisional peer-reviewed toxicity values (PPRTVs) make up the second tier of toxicity values and are developed by the Superfund Health Risk Technical Support Center (STSC). The STSC has assigned a PPRTV to BBP and a "screening value" to DMP, which are available with supporting documentation internally to EPA and on request to registered users. The third tier of EPA's hierarchy of toxicity values, which is a catch-all for "other toxicity values," includes California Environmental Protection Agency Maximum Allowable Dose Levels (MADLs) and Agency for Toxic Substances and Disease Registry (ATSDR) minimal risk levels (MRLs). California has established MADLs for two phthalates, DEHP and DBP; however, the value for DBP is not in the database identified in the EPA procedure (EPA 2003a) for locating other toxicity values, so it has not been included in Table 4-1. ATSDR has established MRLs based on noncancer end points for four phthalates: DEHP (reproduction end point), DBP (developmental end point), DOP (hepatic end point), and DEP (reproductive and hepatic end points). Only the MRL for DEHP applies to the evaluation of chronic exposures, defined by ATSDR as lasting over 365 days. The other MRLs apply to acute exposure (1-7 days) and intermediate exposure (7-364 days).

Only three of the seven phthalates known to cause phthalate syndrome in rats (see Table 3-3) have toxicity values in this hierarchy. Furthermore, the values are based on nonreproductive toxicities with the exception of the ATSDR MRL and the California MADLs for DEHP, and two others (DMP and DEP) are listed that have not been associated with phthalate syndrome. The screening value for DMP developed by EPA's STSC is based on a lowest observed-adverse-effect level associated with increased absolute and relative liver weight and decreased serum and testicular testosterone in weanling male rats. Despite noting the observed lack of adverse effects of DMP on reproductive outcomes or fetal development, the authors of the screening value concluded that "exposure

---

[3]The committee notes that it was not charged with reviewing the basis or adequacy of the values reported in Table 4-1; the committee is simply reporting the current toxicity values for phthalates.

TABLE 4-1 Summary of EPA's Toxicity Values for Phthalates[a]

Phthalate[b] CAS No.	Chronic Oral Reference Dose (mg/kg-d)	Chronic Inhalation Reference Concentration (mg/m³)	Oral Slope Factor (mg/kg-d)⁻¹	Inhalation Unit Risk (μg/m³)⁻¹
DMP CAS 131-11-3	Not available (3/1/1994)[c]	Not available (10/1/1990); EPA contractor updated review (8/2003)	Not available; "D"–not classifiable (2/1/1993), EPA contractor updated review (8/2003)	Not available; "D"–not classifiable (2/1/1993), EPA contractor updated review (8/2003)
DEP CAS 84-66-2	0.8 mg/kg-d; NOAEL, 750 mg/kg-d; uncertainty factor, 1,000 Critical effects from rat subchronic feeding study: decreased growth rate, decreased food consumption, and altered organ weights Low confidence (2/1/1993) EPA contractor updated review (9/2002)	Not available	Not available; "D"–not classifiable (2/1/1993); EPA contractor updated review (9/2002)	Not available; "D"–not classifiable (2/1/1993); EPA contractor updated review (9/2002)
DBP CAS 84-74-2	0.1 mg/kg-d; NOAEL, 125 mg/kg-d; uncertainty factor, 1,000 Critical effect from rat subchronic-to-chronic oral study: increased mortality Low confidence (8/1/1990) EPA contractor updated review (11/2001)	Not available (10/1/1990); EPA contractor updated review (11/2001)	Not available; "D"–not classifiable (2/1/1993); EPA contractor updated review (11/2001)	Not available; "D"–not classifiable (2/1/1993); EPA contractor updated review (11/2001)

(Continued)

TABLE 4-1 Continued

Phthalate[b] CAS No.	Chronic Oral Reference Dose (mg/kg-d)	Chronic Inhalation Reference Concentration (mg/m³)	Oral Slope Factor (mg/kg-d)⁻¹	Inhalation Unit Risk (µg/m³)⁻¹
	Proposed (6/2006): 0.3 mg/kg-d (acute, short term, subchronic, chronic); NOAEL, 30 mg/kg-d; uncertainty factor, 100; critical effect from developmental oral gavage study: developmental (decrease in fetal testosterone)			
BBP CAS 85-68-7	0.2 mg/kg-d: NOAEL, 159 mg/kg-d; uncertainty factor, 1000 Critical effects from 6-mo rat feeding study: significantly increased liver-to-body weight and liver-to-brain weight ratios Low confidence (2/1/1993) EPA contractor updated review (8/2003)	Not available	Not available; "C"–possible human carcinogen (2/1/1993); "qualitative weaknesses of the mononuclear cell leukemia response do not provide a compelling basis to model the dose-response data," EPA contractor updated review (8/2003) *PPRTV*: 1.9×10^{-3} (10/1/2002); pancreatic cancer in male rats	Not available; "C"–possible human carcinogen (2/1/1993); EPA contractor updated review (8/2003)
DEHP CAS 117-81-7	0.02 mg/kg-d; LOAEL 19 mg/kg-d; uncertainty factor, 1000 Critical effect from guinea pig subchronic-to-chronic oral bioassay: increased relative liver weight Medium confidence (5/1/1991)	Not available	1.4×10^{-2}; "B2"–probable human carcinogen (2/1/1993); "orally administered DEHP produced significant dose-related increases in liver tumor responses in rats and mice of both sexes"	Not available

ATSDR MRL:[d] 0.06; uncertainty factor, 100; health end point, reproduction (9/2002)

California EPA:[e] 410 µg/d (adults); 58 µg/d (infant boys, age 29 days-24 months); 20 µg/d (neonatal infant boys, age 0-28 days)

California EPA:[f] Oral CSF, 3×10^{-3}

California EPA:[f] inhalation unit risk, 2.4×10^{-6}

[a]Date of last review is shown in parentheses. Except where otherwise noted, toxicity values are from EPA's IRIS database because these values represent the highest tier in EPA's hierarchy of toxicity values for use at Superfund sites (EPA 2003a).

[b]EPA's IRIS database includes a summary profile of one other phthalate: dimethyl terephthalate (DMT) (CAS 120-61-6; synonym: dimethyl-*p*-phthalate. However, this phthalate is not a diester of 1,2-benzenedicarboxylic acid, so it was not considered by the committee.

[c]EPA's Superfund Health Risk Technical Support Center developed a screening value for DMP (dated September 25, 2007) that probably falls in the third tier of the three-tier hierarchy of toxicity values. It is a subchronic RfD of 0.1 mg/kg-d that incorporates an uncertainty factor of 3,000 and is based on a LOAEL associated with increased absolute and relative liver weight and decreased serum and testicular testosterone in male rats. The authors of the PPRTV documentation concluded that "exposure to multiple phthalate esters in the environment should be taken into consideration when conducting a risk assessment for DMP" (EPA 2007b, p. 15).

[d]Agency for Toxic Substances Disease Registry minimal risk level (ATSDR 2007a). MRLs are also available for three other phthalates to evaluate exposures lasting less than 1 year.

[e]These values are Maximum Allowable Dose Levels (MADLs) for chemicals causing reproductive toxicity. Levels for male children and adolescents can be calculated by application of the default body weights in Title 22, California Code of Regulations, Section 12703(a)(8) to the procedure specified in Title 22, California Code of Regulations, Sections 12801 and 12803. California EPA also established the following MADLs for intravenous exposure: 4,200 µg/d (adults), 600 µg/d (infant boys, age 29 days-24 months), 210 µg/d (neonatal infant boys, age 0-28 days).

[f]California EPA, Office of Environmental Health Hazard Assessment. See OEHHA (2008).

to multiple phthalate esters in the environment should be taken into consideration when conducting a risk assessment for DMP," justifying the statement with the observation that "several phthalate esters may have a common endpoint of toxicity related to developmental and reproductive effects" (EPA 2007b, p. 15).

The hierarchy's entries clearly are largely out of date; any specialized risk assessment of phthalates would presumably consult the recent literature and take account of reproductive toxicity. However, at, for example, a Superfund site, multiple phthalates might be evaluated with the values in Table 4-1.

Special Cases

For some chemicals or chemical classes—such as anticholinesterase-acting pesticides, PCDDs and PCDFs, polychlorinated biphenyls (PCBs), and polycyclic aromatic hydrocarbons—EPA has adopted special approaches that incorporate cumulative risk assessment. Those chemicals are discussed in the section "Current Environmental Protection Agency Cumulative Risk Assessment Examples and Case Studies" below.

When chemicals or exposure circumstances are not suitably matched by any toxicity values in the defined hierarchy of sources discussed above, those performing risk assessments for EPA, such as for Superfund sites, may call on EPA's National Center for Environmental Assessment for assistance (this would presumably occur for phthalates not included in Table 4-1). For others doing risk assessments, evaluation of toxicity values for use in risk assessments is a matter of individual choice. Some toxicity values may be derived by a risk assessor, for example, for assessments appearing in the peer-reviewed literature. In general, the context of the risk assessment dictates the method used to determine the toxicity values.

Risk Characterization of Mixtures: Dose Addition and Independent Action

As pointed out above, many risk assessments performed by using current EPA guidance evaluate simultaneous exposure to multiple chemicals (mixtures), multiple pathways of exposure, multiple routes of exposure, and multiple timeframes of exposure. Before discussing the standard approach to characterizing the risks posed by such exposures, it is helpful to discuss some general concepts of mixture evaluation.

Many terms have been introduced into the literature to describe the combined effect on a particular end point of two or more agents acting simultaneously in comparison with the effect of each agent acting alone. However, the terms have often been used confusingly, contradictorily, inconsistently, or incorrectly (Berenbaum 1989). Some of the confusion and inconsistency in nomenclature stems from attempts to evaluate the combined effects of multiple agents in terms of postulated mechanisms of action rather than in terms of the observed dose-response curves for a given effect. It is unnecessary (although not forbidden) to take account of mechanisms of action in comparing joint effects of multiple exposures with effects of exposures to single agents (Berenbaum 1989); all that is strictly necessary is information on the dose-response relationships for the individual components and information on the dose-response relationships for combinations of those components. That is the position adopted here and in the rest of this report.

When agents in a mixture act together to produce an effect but do not enhance or diminish each other's actions, the resulting mixture is defined to be noninteractive or dose-additive (or concentration-additive when the appropriate exposure measure is concentration). The prototypical noninteractive mixture is a combination of one agent with itself, and the general association between the dose-response relationship of a noninteractive mixture and the dose-response relationships of the individual components has been proved by using this prototype (Berenbaum 1985). The committee notes that the literature can be confusing because of the (implicit or explicit) use of different definitions of noninteraction. However, it is also possible for a particular mixture to be noninteractive according to more than one definition. For example, a mixture could be dose-additive *and* follow the principle of independent action (see next section), which has also on occasion been used to define noninteraction in the literature.

To define dose addition precisely in the general case, consider a mixture with doses d_A of component A, d_B of component B, d_C of component C, and so on; this mixture produces level E of some specific effect. Suppose that the doses of the individual components that each acting alone produce level E of the same specific effect are D_A, D_B, D_C..., where these values are set to infinity if that component does not produce the specific effect at any dose (the case of nonmonotonic dose-response relationships is not considered here but does not present any great difficulties). The mixture is noninteractive, or is dose-additive, if and only if

$$\frac{d_A}{D_A} + \frac{d_B}{D_B} + \frac{d_C}{D_C} + \cdots = 1, \qquad (1)$$

where the sum extends over all components of the mixture. Each combination of doses defines a particular mixture, and the set of all such combinations of doses that provide the same level E of effect is called the isobole for that level of effect.[4] Figure 4-1 gives an example of an isobole for a fixed effect of a two-component mixture and shows synergy, dose addition, and antagonism at different mixture ratios.

---

[4]Geometrically, the isobole is a locally connected hypersurface in the space spanned by dose axes, and the noninteractive mixtures lie on the intersection of this hypersurface with the hyperplane defined by Equation 1.

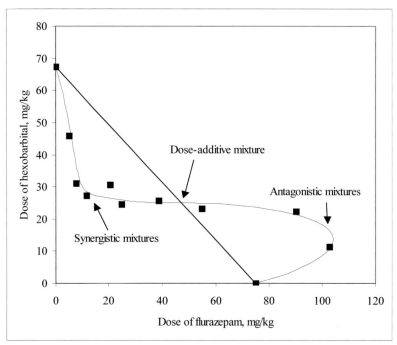

FIGURE 4-1 Isobole for a defined electroencephalographic threshold in anesthesia for mixtures of flurazepam and hexobarbital. Any dose-additive mixture lies on the straight line; the intersection of the line and the isobole indicates the one mixture that is dose-additive for the defined threshold. The solid curve representing the isobole is an ad hoc interpolation between the measured points. Source: Norberg and Wahlström 1988, Table 1. Reprinted with permission; copyright 1988, *Archives Internationales De Pharmacodynamie.*

The statement defining dose addition says nothing about the shapes of the dose-response curves for the individual components, and nothing can be adduced about the dose additivity or non-dose additivity of a mixture from the shapes of the dose-response curves of its components (undocumented statements to the contrary in EPA 2000, Section 4.2.2 and Table B-1, notwithstanding). Several observations about the definition of dose addition are of particular interest.

• First, the dose additivity of a particular mixture does not imply the dose additivity of other mixtures of the same components. Mixtures of the same components may be non-dose additive for different component doses—indeed, may be synergistic (producing an effect larger than expected for dose addition, with the sum of the left side of Equation 1 smaller than unity) at some combinations of component doses, and antagonistic (producing an effect smaller than expected for dose addition, with the sum of the left side of Equation 1 larger than unity) at others. Figure 4-1 provides a striking example of such a situation for a two-component mixture.

- Second, conclusions about dose addition, synergism, or antagonism or more generally about the shape of an isobole may not be the same for different levels of effect even for similar mixture ratios—geometrically, isoboles are not necessarily parallel.
- Third, the doses D_A, D_B, D_C., ... vary with the effect level; indeed, they are just the inverses of the individual dose-response curves of the components. Box 4-2 shows how to derive the dose-additive multiple-dose-response curve for the mixture from the individual dose-response curves of the components.
- Fourth, with the definition of dose addition stipulated by Equation 1, the evaluation of dose-additivity or nonadditivity is a matter entirely for observation using measured dose-response curves; no consideration of mechanism of action is required.
- Fifth, it is not necessary to determine any dose-response curve fully to evaluate additivity or nonadditivity of a mixture at a specific level of effect E. What is required are the doses of the individual components that, acting alone, would give a response level E and the component doses of the mixture that would give a response level E. Then if Equation 1 holds, that mixture is dose-additive at response level E.

Independent Action or Response Addition

An alternative approach to the comparison of the effect of a multicomponent mixture with the effects of individual components is what is often called independent action (also referred to as response addition or Bliss addition). The approach is based on analysis of mechanisms that depend on probabilistically independent events. If $P(A)$ and $P(B)$ are the probabilities for independent events A and B, respectively, to occur, and $Q(A) = 1 - P(A)$ and $Q(B) = 1 - P(B)$ are the corresponding probabilities for events A and B to not occur, then the probability of occurrence of event A or B (that is, occurrence of event A, or event B, or both events) is given by Equation 2, and the probability of nonoccurrence of events A and B is given by Equation 3.

$$P(A \cup B) = P(A) + P(B) - P(A)P(B). \qquad (2)$$

$$Q(A \cup B) = Q(A)Q(B). \qquad (3)$$

Making the "conceptual leap of substituting fractional effect E" of an agent "for probability of occurrence of an event, and the fractional lack of effect

---

BOX 4-2 Derivation of the Dose-Additive Multiple-
Dose-Response Relationship

If the individual dose-response curves for the specific effect considered are $f_A(d)$, $f_B(d)$, $f_C(d)$, ... , respectively, then

$$f_A(D_A) = E \qquad f_B(D_B) = E \qquad f_C(D_C) = E \quad ...$$

$$\text{or} \quad D_A = f_A^{-1}(E) \qquad D_B = f_B^{-1}(E) \qquad D_C = f_C^{-1}(E) \quad ...$$

at effect level E (the second line uses the notation f^{-1} for the inverse function), and there is no requirement for these doses to have the same relative values at different effect levels. Thus Equation 1 may be rewritten as

$$\frac{d_A}{f_A^{-1}(E)} + \frac{d_B}{f_B^{-1}(E)} + \frac{d_C}{f_C^{-1}(E)} + ... = 1.$$

This equation is an implicit dose-additive multiple-dose-response relationship for the mixture in terms of effect level E, the individual doses (d_A, d_B, d_C, ...) of the components, and the individual dose-response relationships (f_A, f_B, f_C, ...) of the components.

(i.e. fractional survival S) for probability of non-occurrence" (Berenbaum 1989) leads to the hypothesis of additivity of effect, or multiplication for survival in the form

$$E_{ab}(d_a, d_b) = E_a(d_a) + E_b(d_b) - E_a(d_a)E_b(d_b)$$

and   (4)

$$S_{ab}(d_a, d_b) = S_a(d_a)S_b(d_b),$$

where $E_a(d_a)$ now represents the fractional effect of agent a at dose d_a and similarly for agent b, and E_{ab} and S_{ab} are the fractional effect and its complement for the mixture of agents a and b at doses d_a and d_b. Some authors use the term *effect addition* when the negative term in the first of Equations 4 is omitted; this is clearly inadequate theoretically for large effects (because it may lead to fractional effects larger than unity), but it is quite adequate for its typical use of combining small effects where the product term is negligible.

Equations 4 and their generalizations to multiple agents define independent action in the same way that Equation 1 defines dose addition. There is no necessary contradiction between the relationships as defined; one, both, or neither may apply to any particular mixture of agents. Contradictions do occur, however, if (as has occurred in the literature; see Berenbaum, 1989 for an extensive review) independent action and noninteraction are assumed to be equivalent, or when synergism and antagonism are defined by deviations from one and inappropriately compared with identical terms defined by deviations from the other.

Empirical Observation vs Mechanistic Inference

With the assumption of dose addition or independent action, the dose-response relationship of a mixture of components may be calculated on the basis of dose-response relationships observed for mixture components. Quite often, the predictions are similar; in other cases, they differ substantially. Where differences arise, they arise from the differences in the mathematical structure of the two models. Neither prediction is guaranteed to correspond to observations. Figure 4-2 provides a hypothetical example in which observations would fall between the predictions of dose addition and independent action; the mixture exhibits synergism with respect to independent action but antagonism with respect to dose addition. Box 4-3 provides the details associated with the hypothetical example represented in Figure 4-2.

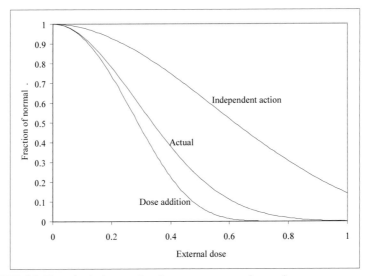

FIGURE 4-2 Hypothetical example of two-component mixture dose-response curve (see Box 4-3). The components are assumed to have the same pharmacokinetics and mechanism of action but different Michaelis-Menten elimination constants and mass-action binding affinity to the same receptor. The fraction of normal response is assumed to be an exponential function of minus the square of the bound fraction of receptors.

BOX 4-3 Hypothetical Example Represented in Figure 4-2

Consider a chemical applied at dose rate d to an organism that has an elimination rate for that chemical that is of Michaelis-Menten form. The concentration C in some target tissue at steady state will then satisfy an equation of the form

$$d = \frac{\lambda C}{k+C},$$

where λ is the maximum elimination rate (so consider dose rates less than λ), and k is the concentration at which the elimination rate is half the maximum. Now suppose that the chemical binds to a receptor according to the law of mass action, so that the fraction of bound receptors is

$$f = \frac{C}{C+Z}$$

for some concentration Z, and the binding to the receptor induces a deviation of some response from normal with magnitude depending on the square of the bound fraction (f), so that the response size is of the form (where the normal response is $R = 1$)

$$R = \exp\left(-hf^2\right)$$

for some constant h.

Now consider two such chemicals with the constants λ, k, Z, and h given by

Parameter	Chemical 1	Chemical 2
λ	1.1	1.4
k	2	0.05
Z	1	0.5
h	75	75

The curves of Figure 4-2 are obtained from a 1:7 mixture of chemical 1 and chemical 2 where chemical 2 and chemical 1 are exact alternative receptor ligands with an effect in a mixture given by

$$f = \frac{C_1 + 2C_2}{1 + C_1 + 2C_2}.$$

The committee emphasizes that dose addition does not imply toxicologic similarity (as defined by EPA 2000), nor does toxicologic similarity imply dose addition, as claimed by EPA (2000); Figure 4-2 is a hypothetical counterexample of the last proposition that shows that dose addition need not apply even to mixtures of components with identical mechanisms of action. Similarly, independent action does not imply, nor is it implied by, different mechanisms for the mixture components. Nor are dose addition and independent action mutually exclusive (see Berenbaum 1989 for counterexamples of these propositions).

Practical Applications, Relative Potencies, and Toxicity Equivalence Factors

Evaluation of any particular mixture of agents requires an empirical determination of how they combine to produce any particular effect. It is generally convenient in performing such evaluations to compare observations against dose addition or independent action, and if the deviations are small enough to be statistically insignificant the mixtures may be considered to exhibit dose addition or independent action for that particular effect at that effect level (many examples of both kinds are known; see Berenbaum 1989 for an extensive review). As pointed out above, dose addition may apply at particular levels of effect (and the same is true of independent action), so a complete evaluation requires examination of all effect levels or at least over the range of effect levels that are of practical importance (effects that might be expected, given the levels of exposure under evaluation). It must be emphasized that any particular finding applies strictly only to the particular effect evaluated; for example, there is nothing to prevent one end point from exhibiting dose addition and another from departing substantially from it at the same dose.

For particular types of mixtures, some plausible assumptions are generally made. Some groups of chemicals may have similar chemical structures and act and be acted on in similar ways in the body. For example, all may be absorbed in the same way (although with quantitative differences in the rate and extent of absorption), and all may be detoxified in the same organ by the same enzyme systems (although with differing V_{max} and k_m for the rate of detoxification). In such circumstances, it is possible and may be plausible to propose—subject to experimental confirmation—that each acts as the same dilution of the other at all doses and in all mixtures. Then, dose addition would apply, and each could be compared directly with some reference agent in the group by using a relative potency that specifies the effective dilution; however, the assumptions, such as similar absorption or detoxification, are not necessarily correct, nor is it necessary that they be satisfied for dose addition to apply. A dose of one agent is then equivalent to a multiple of the dose of another, with the multiple being the same for every dose, so such agents would necessarily have parallel dose-response curves.[5]

Relative potency may, however, differ for different end points. Relative-potency estimates of this nature are used (or are proposed for use) for cancer potency estimates for some chemicals and for noncancer end points for some chemicals, for example, for anticholinesterase agents (see the section "Current EPA Cumulative Risk Assessment Examples and Case Studies" below). Although parallel dose-response curves are necessary for a relative-potency approach to be correctly used, they are not sufficient, because the parallelism of dose-response curves gives no information on the effect of a mixture.

An even more restrictive application of dose addition may be proposed and used in practice, as it has been for the 2,3,7,8-chlorinated dibenzo-*p*-dioxins and -furans and for "dioxin-like" PCB congeners (Van den Berg et al. 2006). For those congeners, a potency estimate, the toxicity equivalence factor (TEF), has been estimated relative to the prototype of the 2,3,7,8-tetrachlorodibenzo-*p*-dioxin group, but this potency is supposed to apply to every end point affected via the aryl hydrocarbon receptor (at least for "dioxin-like" effects in the case of the PCB congeners). By contrast, the less-restrictive relative potencies discussed above may in principle differ for different end points.

Risk Characterization

Practical Risk Characterization for Cancer End Points

For cancer end points, the exposure estimates required to be obtained as described above under "Exposure Assessment" for each receptor evaluated are lifetime average dose rates (expressed in units of milligrams per kilogram per day) or lifetime average exposures (expressed as air or water concentrations). For all pathways of exposure, routes of exposure, and chemicals, individual-chemical risk estimates are obtained by multiplying lifetime average dose rates by the relevant route-specific CSF or multiplying lifetime average exposure by the relevant route-specific unit risks. For brevity, "threshold" carcinogens, for which reference doses and reference concentrations are used in the same manner as noncancer end points, are not addressed here (see EPA 2005a for further guidance). In special circumstances, such as for exposures primarily of young children (EPA 2005b), the standard CSFs may be modified to take account of increased susceptibility of the exposed population.

---

[5]To be consistent with EPA nomenclature, parallel dose-response curves mean that "for equal effects, the dose of one component is a constant [positive] multiple of the dose of a second component" (EPA 2000). The committee added the term *positive* for precision because dose-response curves that are related by a negative multiplier are not considered parallel.

A total cancer risk estimate is then obtained by summing the individual-chemical risk estimates obtained across pathways, routes of exposure, and chemicals. The first two summations, of pathways and routes, are for a single chemical and thus involve no assumptions about interactions between chemicals. The last summation, of chemicals, explicitly incorporates an assumption of independent action (strictly, effect addition). For the end point of interest, lifetime probability of cancer, all carcinogens are treated as having exactly additive effects. For carcinogens at low doses (that is, at lifetime average dose rates low enough for the predicted probability of cancer to be substantially smaller than 0.1—and in practice almost always smaller than 0.001), it is also assumed that the dose-response curve is linear with no threshold. Thus, the effect-addition assumption is in this case also a dose-additive assumption. Because estimated responses are generally sufficiently small for the negative product terms to be negligible in the generalization of Equation 4 to multiple chemicals, independent action and effect addition are equivalent to the accuracies required. Cases in which estimated dose rates are high enough for this not to be true would be treated as obvious emergencies for which any alternative treatment would be unnecessary.

Practical Risk Characterization for Noncancer End Points

For noncancer end points, the exposure estimates required to be obtained as discussed in the section "Exposure Assessment" for each receptor evaluated are average dose rates (expressed in units of milligrams per kilogram per day) or exposures (expressed as air or water concentrations) over a lifetime and over various shorter periods (at any age, but particularly in childhood).

For each chemical, each pathway, and each averaging period, a hazard quotient (HQ) is calculated as

$$HQ = \sum_{routes} \frac{\text{Average dose rate}}{\text{RfD}} \quad \text{or} \quad \frac{\text{Average concentration}}{\text{RfC}}, \quad (5)$$

where the summation is over all routes of exposure, and the RfD or RfC used is appropriate to the averaging period and route or has been adjusted from an alternative averaging period or route to be appropriate. If shorter-term RfD or RfC values (or equivalents from the hierarchic selection of toxicity values) are not available, RfD and RfC values from longer-term exposures may be used for shorter-term exposures, and the resulting HQs are considered likely to be conservative (overestimates).

For each averaging period, an overall summary hazard index (HI) is then calculated as the sum of HQs for each pathway and each chemical, so

$$\text{HI} = \sum_{\text{pathways}} \sum_{\text{chemicals}} \text{HQ.} \tag{6}$$

The summation over chemicals here is explicitly chosen to be a special case of the summation used in the definition of dose addition (compare Equation 1), in which the RfC or RfD used in Equation 5 (and hence in Equation 6) corresponds to a dose rate that has the same effect (namely, no effect) for each chemical. Thus, under the hypothesis of dose addition, if the HI is less than or equal to unity, no effect can be expected from the mixture of chemicals incorporated in the summation. However, the RfC or RfD is not necessarily the largest dose rate or concentration that would result in no effect, so HIs larger than unity cannot necessarily be taken to indicate a larger than zero effect of the mixture under the dose-addition hypothesis, although they are treated as indicators that there is potentially such a nonzero effect.

Thus, if the summary HI is less than or equal to unity, there is unlikely to be an appreciable risk of deleterious effects, and the analysis is usually complete. If the summary HI is larger than unity, further analysis may be performed that takes account of "effect" and "mechanism of action" in an attempt to determine whether application of dose addition to all the chemicals simultaneously is justifiable or to determine whether the RfD or RfC used in evaluating the summation is appropriate for any particular common effect or mechanism (see the section "Empirical Observation vs Mechanistic Inference" above).

EPA guidance on segregation of chemicals by effect is shown in Box 4-4. The guidance states further that "if one of the effect-specific hazard indices exceeds unity, consideration of the mechanism of action might be warranted. A strong case is required, however, to indicate that two compounds which produce adverse effects on the same organ system (e.g., liver), although by different mechanisms, should not be treated as dose additive. Any such determination should be reviewed by ECAO [Environmental Criteria and Assessment Office in EPA's Office of Health and Environmental Assessment]" (EPA 1989a, p. 8-14).

It is further pointed out that obtaining the information required to segregate chemicals by effect or mechanism of action is difficult to locate (see Box 4-5 below).

Furthermore, "if there are specific data germane to the assumption of dose-additivity (e.g., if two compounds are present at the same site and it is known that the combination is five times more toxic than the sum of toxicities for the two compounds), then modify the development of the hazard index accordingly. Refer to the EPA (1986) mixtures guidelines for discussion of a hazard index equation that incorporates quantitative interaction data. If data on chemical interactions are available, but are not adequate to support a quantitative assessment, note the information in the 'assumptions' being documented for the site risk assessment" (EPA 1989a, pp. 8-14).

BOX 4-4 Procedure for Segregation of Hazard Indexes by Effect

Segregation of hazard indices requires identification of the major effects of each chemical, including those seen at higher doses than the critical effect (e.g., the chemical may cause liver damage at a dose of 100 mg/kg-day and neurotoxicity at a dose of 250 mg/kg-day). Major effect categories include neurotoxicity, developmental toxicity, reproductive toxicity, immunotoxicity, and adverse effects by target organ (i.e., hepatic, renal, respiratory, cardiovascular, gastrointestinal, hematological, musculoskeletal, and dermal/ocular effects). Although higher exposure levels may be required to produce adverse health effects other than the critical effect, the RfD can be used as the toxicity value for each effect category as a conservative and simplifying step.

Source: EPA 1989a.

BOX 4-5 Information Sources for Segregation of Hazard Indexes

Of the available information sources, the ATSDR Toxicological Profiles are well suited in format and content to allow a rapid determination of additional health effects that may occur at exposure levels higher than those that produce the critical effect. Readers should be aware that the ATSDR definitions of exposure durations are somewhat different than EPA's and are independent of species; acute—up to 14 days; intermediate—more than 14 days to 1 year; chronic—greater than 1 year. IRIS contains only limited information on health effects beyond the critical effect, and EPA criteria documents and HEAs, HEEPs, and HEEDs may not systematically cover all health effects observed at doses higher [than] those associated with the most sensitive effects.

Source: EPA 1989a.

Special Considerations in Practical Risk Characterizations

As pointed out above, some groups of chemicals are treated specially by using relative-potency or TEF approaches; these are discussed further in the section "Current EPA Cumulative Risk Assessment Examples and Case Studies" below. Some mixtures, such as Aroclors (PCB mixtures), may be treated as individual chemicals in toxicity assessments because they have been tested in toxicity studies. However, it is unlikely that the precise mixtures tested (and there may be some doubt as to their characterization in any case) will ever be what receptors are exposed to after transport through the environment, so actual exposures are likely to be to mixtures with congener or other component profiles differing from those tested. There are also situations in which the risk assessments required do not correspond completely to the "typical" assessment described here, such as nationwide evaluations of cumulative and aggregate exposures to pesticides (*cumulative* refers to the multiple-chemical nature of the assessment and *aggregate* to the multiple pathways of exposure).

Summary of Current Risk-Assessment Approaches

In summary, the usual approach to EPA-style risk assessments for non-cancer end points is initially "dose-additive" for all chemicals, partly to ensure an initial conservative assessment. Later, if such a conservative approach does not suffice, the dose-addition approach is applied independently to subsets of chemicals with the same end point or mechanism, where *mechanism* is not well defined. For cancer end points, the usual approach of summing risk estimates for all chemicals is both response-additive and dose-additive because the two are equivalent when the standard low-dose linear hypothesis is used.[6] In every case, direct information on any particular mixture that contradicts the hypothesis of dose addition will override the default approach.

THE EVOLUTION OF GUIDANCE ON CUMULATIVE
RISK ASSESSMENT

Table 4-2 summarizes the evolution of EPA guidance (or, for the International Life Sciences Institute document, in cooperation with EPA) on cumulative risk assessment. Undoubtedly, other documents have influenced the practice of cumulative risk assessment, but the committee believes that those cited here have been the primary sources for EPA consideration of cumulative risk assessment. Table 4-2 summarizes the stated purpose of the guidance, the definitions of *cumulative* adopted in the guidance document, and the default approach taken for evaluation of cumulative risks posed by mixtures of chemicals and other stressors when there is no direct information on the particular (or sufficiently similar) mixtures (so that the effect of the mixture has to be estimated from measured effects of individual components). As far as possible, the committee has quoted the documents or relevant memoranda accompanying the documents on their release for the summaries. At times, that proved difficult because there may be more than one statement or definition, and the default approach may not have been explicitly stated. The "Default approach" column of the table highlights some statements made in the guidance about the conditions required for dose addition or independent action.

---

[6]For brevity, "threshold" carcinogens were not addressed here.

TABLE 4-2 Summary of Stated Purposes of Guidance Documents, Definition of *Cumulative* in the Context of Risk Assessment, and the Default Approach Taken to the Toxicity of Mixtures of Chemicals

Document Title, Author Agency, Date	Stated Purpose	Definition of *Cumulative*	Default Approach
Guidelines for the Health Risk Assessment of Chemical Mixtures, EPA/630/R-98/002, September 1986, Risk Assessment Forum, also published 51FR34014-34025	"Generate a consistent Agency approach for evaluating data on the chronic and subchronic effects of chemical mixtures" (EPA 1986, p. 1)	Not defined	Although all authorities cited adopted dose-additive models, "dose additive models are not the most biologically plausible approach if the compounds do not have the same mode of toxicologic action," and the recommendation was that "depending on the nature of the risk assessment and the available information on modes of action and patterns of joint action, the ... most reasonable additive model should be used." (Dose addition and independent action are the only alternatives discussed.) Later, however, a hazard-index approach (dose addition) is recommended for systemic toxicants, although "since the assumption of dose addition is most properly applied to compounds that induce the same effect by similar modes of action, a separate hazard index should be generated for each end point of concern." (EPA 1986, pp. 8-9)
Technical Support Document on Risk Assessment of Chemical Mixtures, EPA/600/8-90/064, November 1988, Office of Research and Development	Supplement to 1986 guidelines	Limited to mixtures of chemicals	None.

(Continued)

TABLE 4-2 Continued

Document Title, Author Agency, Date	Stated Purpose	Definition of *Cumulative*	Default Approach
Risk Assessment Guidance for Superfund, Volume 1, Human Health Evaluation Manual (Part A), Interim Final, EPA/540/1-89/002, December 1989	"Developed to be used in the remedial investigation/feasibility study (RI/FS) process at Superfund sites, although the analytical framework and specific methods described in the manuals may also be applicable to other assessments of hazardous wastes and hazardous materials" (EPA 1989a, p. xv)	Not defined; cites to 1986 guidelines for using dose addition for "aggregate" risks of multiple chemicals; "although the calculation procedures differ for carcinogenic and noncarcinogenic effects, both sets of procedures assume dose additivity in the absence of information on specific mixtures" (EPA 1989a, pp. 8-12) Chemicals and radiation only	Default is dose addition; hazard quotients are summed to produce a hazard index (HI). "If the HI is greater than unity...it would be appropriate to segregate the compounds by effect and by mechanism of action." Furthermore, "if one of the effect-specific hazard indices exceeds unity, consideration of the mechanism of action might be warranted. A strong case is required, however, to indicate that two compounds which produce adverse effects on the same organ system (e.g., liver), although by different mechanisms, should not be treated as dose additive." (EPA 1989a, p. 8-14)
Guidance on Cumulative Risk Assessment, Part I Planning and Scoping, EPA Science Policy Council, July 3, 1997; memo from EPA administrator, July 3, 1997, quoted	"This guidance directs each office to take into account cumulative risk issues in scoping and planning major risk assessments and to consider a broader scope that integrates multiple sources, effects, pathways, stressors and populations for cumulative risk analyses in all cases for which relevant data are available." (EPA 1997a, p. 1)	"Adverse health and ecological effects from synthetic chemicals, radiation, and biological stressors," "social, economic, behavioral or psychological stressors that may contribute to adverse health effects," including "existing health condition, anxiety, nutritional status, crime, and congestion." (EPA 1997b, p. 2)	"Due to the current state of the practice and limited data, the aggregation of risks may often be based on a default assumption of additivity." (EPA 1997b, p. 3) (there is no definition of *additivity*.)
A Framework for Cumulative Risk Assessment, ILSI Risk Science Institute Workshop Report (1999)	"The goal of this project is to develop a framework that can be used to guide the conduct of cumulative risk assessments." (ILSI 1999, p. 2)	Implicitly examined only multiple chemical exposures	No default is specified, although the text may imply some sort of unspecified additivity at low dose.

Supplementary Guidance for Conducting Health Risk Assessment of Chemical Mixtures, EPA/630/R-00/002, August 2000; Risk Assessment Forum	"This document describes more detailed procedures for chemical mixture assessment using data on the mixture of concern, data on a toxicologically similar mixture, and data on the mixture component chemicals." (EPA 2000, p. xiv) Examines only chemical mixtures, intended as only a component of a cumulative assessment as described by EPA 1997b (above)	Default of hazard index or relative potency for "toxicologically similar" components, independent action for "toxicologically independent" components, interaction hazard index for "interactions" "In practice, because of the common lack of information on mode of action and pharmacokinetics, the requirement of toxicologic similarity is usually relaxed to that of similarity of target organs (U.S. EPA, 1989a)." (EPA 2000, p. 80) Citation is to guidance listed above.
Guidance on Cumulative Risk Assessment of Pesticide Chemicals That Have a Common Mechanism of Toxicity, EPA Office of Pesticide Programs, January 14, 2002	"This document provides guidance to OPP [Office of Pesticide Programs] scientists for evaluating and estimating the potential human risks associated with such multichemical and multipathway exposures to pesticides." (EPA 2002, p. ii) "This document provides guidance to OPP scientists for evaluating and estimating the potential human risks associated with such multichemical and multipathway exposures to pesticides. This process is referred to as cumulative risk assessment." (EPA 2002, p. ii)	"A cumulative risk assessment begins with the identification of a group of chemicals, a Common Mechanism Group (CMG), that induce a common toxic effect by a common mechanism of toxicity." (EPA 2002, p. iii) EPA here assumes that identification of a CMG implies dose addition for its member chemicals, so dose addition is the only possibility considered. It is also asserted (incorrectly) that "dose addition requires a constant proportionality among the effectiveness of the chemicals." (EPA 2002, p. 31)

(Continued)

TABLE 4-2 Continued

Document Title, Author Agency, Date	Stated Purpose	Definition of *Cumulative*	Default Approach
Framework for Cumulative Risk Assessment, EPA/630/P-02/001F, May 2003, Risk Assessment Forum	"Immediately offers a basic structure and provides starting principles for EPA's cumulative risk assessments" (EPA 2003b, p. 5) "Offers the basic principles around which to organize a more definitive set of cumulative risk assessment guidance" (EPA 2003b, p. 5)	"Cumulative Risk: The combined risks from aggregate exposures to multiple agents or stressors." (EPA 2003b, p. 6) "Aggregate exposure: The combined exposure of an individual (or defined population) to a specific agent or stressor via relevant routes, pathways, and sources." (EPA 2003b, p. 7)	No explicit default; refers to previous documents, particularly EPA (2000), in which defaults are specified.
Concepts, Methods and Data Sources for Cumulative Health Risk Assessment of Multiple Chemicals, Exposures and Effects: A Resource Document. EPA/600/R-06/013F, August 2007, EPA, National Center for Environmental Assessment, Cincinnati, OH	"This current report serves as a resource document for identifying specific elements of and approaches for implementing cumulative risk assessments. This report is not a regulatory document and is not guidance but rather a presentation of concepts, methods and data sources." (EPA 2007g, p. xvii)	"The Framework defines cumulative risk as the combined risks from aggregate exposures (i.e., multiple route exposures) to multiple agents or stressors, where agents or stressors may include chemicals, as well as biological or physical agents (e.g., noise, nutritional status), or the absence of a necessity such as habitat (U.S. EPA, 2003a). Cumulative risk assessment, then, is an analysis, characterization and possible quantification of the combined risks to health or the environment from multiple agents or stressors." (EPA 2007g, p. xxi), citation in the quote is to the framework listed above.	No explicit default; refers to previous documents, particularly EPA (2000), in which defaults are specified.

CURRENT ENVIROMENTAL PROTECTION AGENCY EXAMPLES AND CASE STUDIES OF CUMULATIVE RISK ASSESSMENT

Cumulative risk assessment is not new, although development and application of relevant EPA guidance continues to evolve (see, for example, EPA 2007g). EPA's IRIS database includes toxicity values for chemical mixtures, such as coke-oven emissions, diesel-engine exhaust, PCBs, xylene isomers, a 2,4- and 2,6-dinitrotoluene mixture, and a 2,4- and 2,6-toluene diisocyanate mixture. In addition, Table 4-3 highlights recent applications of cumulative risk assessment to evaluate human exposure to chemicals. The following sections provide more detailed descriptions of two EPA programs that involve cumulative evaluations of pesticides and air toxics.

Aggregate and Cumulative Assessments of Pesticides

EPA's Office of Pesticide Programs implements a two-stage assessment process for groups of pesticides that have a common mechanism of toxicity. First, an aggregate assessment that considers all pathways and routes of exposure of each member of the group is completed (EPA 2008d,e); depending on the results, risk-reduction actions may be taken. Then a cumulative assessment considers exposure of and risks to all members of the group; additional risk-reduction steps may be taken on the basis of the results. Risk-reduction actions include elimination or restriction of pesticide uses.

Cumulative risk assessments of pesticides with a common mechanism of toxicity involve extensive dose-response modeling for each pesticide, which provides the relative potencies used in the dose-additivity-based cumulative method for common-mechanism pesticides (EPA 2002). Such risk assessments also involve a multicomponent exposure assessment (EPA 2002). Dietary exposures are estimated from nationally representative dietary and pesticide-residue surveys. Drinking-water exposures and residential and nonoccupational pesticide uses are estimated by region to reflect variations in agriculture, pest pressures, and home and other pesticide uses. The datasets are compiled into an individual-level daily-exposure estimate over the course of a year. For the risk characterization, relevant durations of exposure are defined, and rolling-average exposures to individuals are developed on the basis of the daily-exposure estimates (EPA 2002). As implied in the descriptions of dose-response and exposure-assessment procedures, cumulative risk assessments of common-mechanism pesticides involve consideration of the timing and duration of exposures and the timing of onset and duration of health effects and recovery (EPA 2002).

TABLE 4-3 Summary of Cumulative Human Risk Assessment Applications to Evaluation of Chemical Exposures[a]

Chemical Mixture	Cumulative Risk Assessment Approach	References
Asbestos fibers	Asbestos includes various naturally occurring silicate fibers, and their cancer potency may vary as a function of fiber type and size. Therefore, EPA developed draft guidance, currently undergoing review by its Science Advisory Board, that provides an approach for quantifying differences in cancer potency among fiber types (amphibole or chrysotile) and particle sizes (length and width).	EPA 2008f
Carcinogenic polycyclic aromatic hydrocarbons	EPA classifies benzo[a]pyrene (B[a]P) and six other polycyclic aromatic hydrocarbons (PAHs) as B2 carcinogens. Results are consistent among cancer bioassays involving B[a]P and these PAHs; however, insufficient data are available to derive cancer slope factors for all these PAHs. Also, although these PAHs may cause cancer by the same mechanism as B[a]P, they appear to be less potent. EPA developed a relative-potency approach to estimate cancer risk associated with these PAHs by comparing PAH cancer potencies, using skin tumorogenicity bioassays, and quantifying "order of magnitude" relative potency factors (RPFs) for the six carcinogenic PAHs on the basis of comparison with the index chemical, B[a]P. This RPF approach can be used to evaluate PAH mixtures as they occur in the environment, with proportions depending on source, age of release, and environmental conditions. EPA is re-evaluating the toxicity of B[a]P and recently presented preliminary analyses in which EPA defined 26 PAHs, instead of the current six, with adequate data for RPF derivation.	EPA 1993b; Carlson-Lynch et al. 2007
Dioxin-like chemicals	People are exposed to 2,3,7,8-tetrachlorodibenzo-p-dioxin (2,3,7,8-TCDD, or "dioxin") and other 2,3,7,8-chlorinated dioxin congeners and dioxin-like compounds as complex mixtures. Seven dioxin, 10 furan, and 12 polychlorinated biphenyl (PCB) congeners may exert toxic effects through the same mechanism of action as 2,3,7,8-TCDD, namely, binding to the aryl hydrocarbon receptor (AhR), a cellular protein. A toxic equivalence (TEQ) approach has been developed to estimate risk associated with 2,3,7,8-TCDD and other dioxin-like congeners. The approach applies to AhR-mediated effects, assuming a model of dose addition. Each dioxin-like congener has been assigned a toxic equivalence factor (TEF) to represent the fractional toxicity of the congener relative to that of 2,3,7,8-TCDD. TEFs are used to transform concentrations of individual dioxin-like congeners into an equivalent concentration of 2,3,7,8-TCDD, as determined by the equation $$TEQ = \sum_{i \in PCDDs} [(C_i)(TEF_i)] + \sum_{i \in PCDFs} [(C_i)(TEF_i)] + \sum_{i \in PCBs} [(C_i)(TEF_i)],$$	EPA 1987, 1989b; Van den Berg et al. 1998, 2006

where TEQ = equivalent TCDD concentration, TEF_i = toxic equivalency factor for congener i, and C_i = concentration of congener i.

This TEQ estimate is combined with toxicity data on 2,3,7,8-TCDD to quantify risk posed by exposure to dioxin-like congener mixtures.

Polychlorinated biphenyls	Commercial PCB mixtures released into the environment may be altered as a result of environmental processes, such as partitioning, transformation, and bioaccumulation through the food chain. Therefore, EPA recommends an approach to assess cancer risk associated with exposure to PCBs that accounts for different PCB mixtures typically found in environmental media. Cancer studies to date suggest that more highly chlorinated, less volatile congeners are associated with greater cancer risk. Those congeners tend to persist in the environment in soil and sediment and to bioaccumulate in biota. More volatile, less chlorinated congeners that partition into air or surface water are more likely to be metabolized and eliminated than highly chlorinated congeners. Therefore, EPA recommends using the noncancer medium or exposure medium as an indicator of the cancer potency of a PCB mixture. For noncancer effects, EPA has developed reference doses for two commercial PCB mixtures (Aroclor 1016 and Aroclor 1254), which account for the toxicity of the mixtures but not necessarily how they might have changed after release into the environment.	EPA 1996a,b,c; EPA 1997c
Petroleum hydrocarbon fractions	The composition of petroleum products changes after release into the environment. For that reason, use of toxicity data on whole products may be appropriate for fresh spills but not for older spills that have had time to weather. Alternatively, evaluating only a subset of individual chemicals in a mixture, such as carcinogenic PAHs and benzene, might not account for toxicity associated with the rest of the mixture. Therefore, a fraction-based approach was devised that consists of dividing petroleum mixtures into fractions and assigning physical and chemical properties and toxicity values to each fraction. This approach accounts for environmental weathering of spilled product and is a practical alternative to evaluation of hundreds of individual petroleum chemicals. Furthermore, data on toxicity and fate and transport properties needed for assessing health risk are not available for many petroleum hydrocarbons.	MADEP 2002, 2003; Edwards et al. 1997; Gustafson et al. 1997
ATSDR interaction profiles	The Comprehensive Environmental Response, Compensation, and Liability Act (CERCLA) directs ATSDR, where feasible, to develop methods for determining the health effects of substances in combination with other substances with which they are commonly found. Exposure to two or more chemicals is common at hazardous-waste sites that ATSDR evaluates. Therefore, ATSDR developed a chemical-mixtures program in response to the CERCLA directive, including identification of mixtures of highest concern for pubic health and publication of final interaction profiles that evaluate toxicity data on a whole mixture, where available, and otherwise rely on mostly binary data relevant to the	ATSDR 2004, 2007b

(Continued)

TABLE 4-3 Continued

Chemical Mixture	Cumulative Risk Assessment Approach	References
	joint toxic action of chemicals in the mixture. ATSDR has completed profiles for the following mixtures: (1) arsenic, cadmium, chromium, and lead; (2) benzene, toluene, ethylbenzene, and xylenes; (3) lead, manganese, zinc, and copper; (4) persistent chemicals found in breast milk; (5) persistent chemicals found in fish; (6) 1,1,1-trichloroethane, 1,1-dichloroethane, trichloroethylene, and tetrachloroethylene; (7) cesium, cobalt, PCBs, strontium, and trichloroethylene; (8) arsenic, hydrazines, jet fuels, strontium-90, and trichloroethylene; (9) cyanide, fluoride, nitrate, uranium; (10) atrazine, deethylatrazine, diazinon, nitrate, simazine; and (11) chlorpyrifos, lead, mercury, and methylmercury.	
Disinfection byproducts	People are exposed simultaneously to disinfection byproducts in drinking water. EPA developed an approach to cumulative risk assessment of disinfection-byproduct mixtures that requires exposure modeling and physiologically based pharmacokinetic modeling combined with the use of cumulative relative potency factors (CRPFs). The use of CRPFs provides multiple-route, chemical-mixture risk estimates based on total absorbed doses.	EPA 2003c; Teuschler et al. 2004

[a]Pesticides and air toxics are described in detail in text.

No new regulatory actions were needed on the basis of EPA's recent cumulative assessment of 10 *N*-methyl carbamate pesticides because actions taken on the basis of aggregate assessments of the individual pesticides had achieved necessary risk reductions (EPA 2008g). For example, all domestic uses of carbofuran were deemed ineligible for reregistration, given the findings of its aggregate assessment. All U.S. uses of carbofuran will be canceled (EPA 2007c).

National Air Toxics Assessment

The National Air Toxics Assessment (NATA) is a national assessment of health risks associated with inhalation of 33 hazardous air pollutants (air toxics) and diesel particulate matter (qualitative assessment only). Assessment results are disseminated online for the public and used to inform the air-toxics program in priority-setting, air-pollution trends assessment, research, and planning (EPA 2007d).

The NATA estimates concurrent exposures to the selected chemicals at the census-tract, county or state level at a selected time (EPA 2006). The cumulative methods applied for the NATA are dose addition and independent action. The common noncancer health effect of concern is respiratory irritation (irritation of the lining of the respiratory system), and single-chemical HQs of respiratory irritants are added to yield a "respiratory hazard index" (dose addition). For the carcinogens, lifetime cancer risk estimates for inhalation exposures are added (independent action but also in effect dose addition because of the assumed dose-response linearity) (EPA 2007e).

More than 25 million people live in census tracts where air pollutants contribute to upper-bound estimates of more than 10 in 1 million increment in lifetime cancer risk. The most important carcinogens that are known to contribute to the estimated excess risks are benzene and chromium (EPA 2007f).

STRENGTHS AND WEAKNESSES OF CURRENT APPROACHES OR PRACTICES

Having reviewed the current cumulative risk assessment practices and approaches, the committee has made the following observations:

- EPA has been addressing cumulative impact and risk under various legal and regulatory authorities.
- Various offices and organizations in the EPA have devoted considerable resources to developing concepts and guidance regarding cumulative risk assessment.
- In cumulative risk assessments of human health effects, there is a reliance on dose addition as the default approach.

- Current practices focus on well-defined mixtures of chemical stressors to which simultaneous (or concurrent) exposures occur.

In its *Framework for Cumulative Risk Assessment* (EPA 2003b), EPA has developed an appropriately broad definition of cumulative risk assessment and identified multiple approaches to the conduct of such assessments. EPA, through its various offices, has accrued substantial practical experience with cumulative risk assessment. However, the assessments conducted to date have been of well-defined groups of chemicals to which simultaneous exposure occurs. Chemicals are grouped according to a common mechanism of toxic action or end point and specific exposure situations, such as a hazardous-waste site or spill or presence in food or water. Therefore, although multiple methods are available, EPA has used only a few of them in practice. And despite recognition of nonchemical stressors as potentially important contributors to cumulative risk, nonchemical stressors are rarely addressed or evaluated.

APPLICATION TO PHTHALATES

EPA clearly has given considerable thought to cumulative risk assessment and has produced substantial guidance on it. On the basis of that guidance, a mixture of phthalates should be included in a cumulative assessment based on "toxicologic similarity" (see Chapter 3). However, there may be inconsistencies in how different offices in EPA would perform risk assessments, the available IRIS toxicity values do not incorporate the relevant end points that would suggest toxicologic similarity, and some of the guidance is pulling in different directions in that toxicologic similarity is largely undefined. A sufficiently detailed examination of the toxicologic profiles and mechanisms of action of the individual phthalates would find distinct differences in end points affected or the degree to which specific end points are affected and in detailed mechanisms of action, so toxicologic similarity would be ambiguous.

The following chapter examines the evaluation of phthalate mixtures in more detail and provides practical approaches to the examination of phthalates mixtures in particular and other mixtures in general.

REFERENCES

ATSDR (Agency for Toxic Substances and Disease Registry). 2004. Guidance Manual for the Assessment of Joint Toxic Action of Chemical Mixtures. U.S. Department of Health and Human Services, Public Health Service, Agency for Toxic Substances and Disease Registry. May 2004 [online]. Available: http://www.atsdr. cdc.gov/interactionprofiles/ipga.html [accessed July 22, 2008].

ATSDR (Agency for Toxic Substances and Disease Registry). 2007a. Minimum Risk Levels (MRLs) for Hazardous Substances, November 2007 [online]. Available: http://www.atsdr.cdc.gov/mrls/ [accessed June 16, 2008].

ATSDR (Agency for Toxic Substances and Disease Registry). 2007b. Final Interaction Profiles [online]. Availble: http://www.atsdr.cdc.gov/interactionprofiles/ [accessed June 16, 2008].

Berenbaum, M.C. 1985. The expected effect of a combination of agents: The general solution. J. Theor. Biol. 114(3):413-431.

Berenbaum, M.C. 1989. What is synergy? Pharmacol. Rev. 41(2):93-141.

Carlson-Lynch, H., J. Stickney, P. McClure, M. Gehlhaus, and L. Flowers. 2007. Proposed Derivation of Relative Potency Factors (RPFs) for Individual Polycyclic Aromatic Hydrocarbons and Characterization of Uncertainty. Abstract M3-E5. Presented at the Society for Risk Analysis Annual Meeting 2007-Risk 007: Agents of Analysis, December 9-12, 2007, San Antonio, TX [online]. Available: http://birenheide.com/sra/2007AM/program/singlesession.php3?sessid=M3-E [accessed July 15, 2008].

Edwards, D.A., M.D. Andriot, M.A. Amoruso, A.C. Tummey, C.J. Bevan, A. Tveit, L.A. Hayes, S.H. Youngren, and D.V. Nakles. 1997. Development of Fraction Specific Reference Doses (RfDs) and Reference Concentrations (RfCs) for Total Petroleum Hydrocarbons (TPH). Total Petroleum Hydrocarbon Criteria Working Group Series, Vol. 4. Amherst, MA: Amherst Scientific Publishers [online]. Available: http://www.aehs.com/publications/catalog/contents/Volume4.pdf [accessed July 23, 2008].

EPA (U.S. Environmental Protection Agency). 1986. Guidelines for the Health Risk Assessment of Chemical Mixtures. EPA/630/R-98/002. Risk Assessment Forum, U.S. Environmental Protection Agency, Washington, DC. September 1986 [online]. Available: http://www.epa.gov/ncea/raf/pdfs/chem_mix/chemmix_1986.pdf [accessed July 23, 2008].

EPA (U.S. Environmental Protection Agency). 1987. Interim Procedures for Estimating Risks Associated with Exposures to Mixtures of Chlorinated Dibenzo-*p*-Dioxins and -Dibenzofurans (CDDs and CDFs). EPA/625/3-87/012. Risk Assessment Forum, U.S. Environmental Protection Agency, Washington, DC. March 1987.

EPA (U.S. Environmental Protection Agency). 1989a. Risk Assessment Guidance for Superfund, Volume I. Human Health Evaluation Manual (Part A). Interim Final. EPA/540/1-89/002. PB90-155581. Office of Emergency and Remedial Response, U.S. Environmental Protection Agency, Washington, DC. December 1989 [online]. Available: http://rais.ornl.gov/homepage/HHEMA.pdf [accessed July 22, 2008].

EPA (U.S. Environmental Protection Agency). 1989b. Interim Procedures for Estimating Risks Associated with Exposures to Mixtures of Chlorinated Dibenzo-*p*-Dioxins and -Dibenzofurans (CDDs and CDFs) and 1989 Update. EPA/625/3-89/016. Risk Assessment Forum, U.S. Environmental Protection Agency, Washington, DC. March 1989.

EPA (U.S. Environmental Protection Agency). 1992. Guidelines for Exposure Assessment. EPA/600/Z-92/001. Risk Assessment Forum, U.S. Environmental Protection Agency, Washington, DC. May 1992 [online]. Available: http://rais.ornl.gov/homepage/GUIDELINES_EXPOSURE_ASSESSMENT.pdf [accessed July 22, 2008].

EPA (U.S. Environmental Protection Agency). 1993a. Use of IRIS Values in Superfund Risk Assessment. OSWER Directive 9285.7-16. Memorandum to Directors, Waste Management Division Region I, IV, VII, VIII, Director, Emergency and Remedial Response Division Region II, Directors, Hazardous Waste Management Division

Regions III, VI, IX, and Directors, Hazardous Waste Division, Region X, from William H. Farland, Director, Office of Health and Environmental Assessment, Henry L. Longest II, Director, Office of Emergency and Remedial Response, U.S Environmental Protection Agency, Washington, DC. December 21, 1993 [online]. Available http://www.epa.gov/oswer/riskassessment/pdf/irismemo.pdf [accessed May 13, 2008].

EPA (U.S. Environmental Protection Agency). 1993b. Provisional Guidance for Quantitative Risk Assessment of Polycyclic Aromatic Hydrocarbons. EPA/600/R-93/089. Office of Research and Development, U.S. Environmental Protection Agency, Washington, DC. July 1993 [online]. Available: http://www.epa.gov/oswer/risk assessment/pdf/1993_epa_600_r-93_c89.pdf [accessed June 10, 2008].

EPA (U.S. Environmental Protection Agency). 1996a. Aroclor 1016 (CASRN 12674-11-2). Integrated Risk Information System, U.S. Environmental Protection Agency [online]. Available: http://www.epa.gov/ncea/iris/subst/0462.htm [accessed July 22, 2008].

EPA (U.S. Environmental Protection Agency). 1996b. Aroclor 1254 (CASRN 11097-69-1). Integrated Risk Information System, U.S. Environmental Protection Agency [online]. Available: http://www.epa.gov/ncea/iris/subst/0389.htm [accessed July 22, 2008].

EPA (U.S. Environmental Protection Agency). 1996c. PCBs: Cancer Dose-Response Assessment and Application to Environmental Mixtures. EPA/600/P-96/001F. National Center for Environmental Assessment, Office of Research and Development, U.S. Environmental Protection Agency, Washington, DC. September 1996 [online]. Available: http://www.epa.gov/pcb/pubs/pcb.pdf [accessed June 10, 2008].

EPA (U.S. Environmental Protection Agency). 1997a. Cumulative Risk Assessment Guidance-Phase I Planning and Scoping. Memorandum to Assistant Administrators, General Counsel, Inspector General, Associate Administrators, Regional Administrators, Staff Office Directors, from Carol M. Browner, Administrator, and Fred Hansen, Deputy Administrator, U.S. Environmental Protection Agency. July 3, 1997 [online]. Available: http://www.epa.gov/OSA/spc/pdfs/cumulrisk.pdf [accessed July 23, 2008].

EPA (U.S. Environmental Protection Agency). 1997b. Guidance on Cumulative Risk Assessment. Part 1. Planning and Scoping. Science Policy Council, U.S. Environmental Protection Agency, Washington, DC. July 3, 1997 [online]. Available: http://www.epa.gov/OSA/spc/pdfs/cumrisk2.pdf [accessed July 22, 2008].

EPA (U.S. Environmental Protection Agency). 1997c. Polychlorinated Biphenyls (PCBs) (CASRN 1336-36-3). Integrated Risk Information System, U.S. Environmental Protection Agency [online]. Available: http://www.epa.gov/ncea/iris/subst/ 0294.htm [accessed July 22, 2008].

EPA (U.S. Environmental Protection Agency). 2000. Supplementary Guidance for Conducting Health Risk Assessment of Chemical Mixtures. EPA/630/R-00/002. Risk Assessment Forum, U.S. Environmental Protection Agency, Washington, DC. August 2000 [online]. Available: http://www.epa.gov/NCEA/raf/pdfs/chem_mix/ chem_mix_08_2001.pdf [accessed June 10, 2008].

EPA (U.S. Environmental Protection Agency). 2001. Risk Assessment Guidance for Superfund, Volume 3- Part A: Process for Conducting Probabilistic Risk Assessment. EPA 540-R-02-002. Office of Emergency and Remedial Response, U.S. Environmental Protection Agency, Washington, DC. December 2001 [online]. Available: http://www.epa.gov/oswer/riskassessment/rags3adt/ [accessed July 22, 2008].

EPA (U.S. Environmental Protection Agency). 2002. Guidance on Cumulative Risk Assessment of Pesticide Chemicals That Have a Common Mechanism of Toxicity. Office of Pesticide Programs, U.S. Environmental Protection Agency, Washington, DC. January 14, 2002 [online]. Available: http://www.epa.gov/oppfead1/trac/ science/cumulative_guidance.pdf [accessed June 10, 2008].

EPA (U.S. Environmental protection Agency). 2003a. Human Health Toxicity Values in Superfund Risk Assessments. OSWER Directive 9285.7-53. Memorandum to Superfund National Policy Managers, Regions 1 - 10, from Michael B. Cook, Director, Office of Superfund Remediation and Technology Innovation, Washington, DC. December 5, 2003 [online]. Available: http://www.epa.gov/oswer/riskassess ment/pdf/hhmemo.pdf [accessed May 13, 2008].

EPA (U.S. Environmental Protection Agency). 2003b. Framework for Cumulative Risk Assessment. EPA/630/P-02/001F. Risk Assessment Forum, U.S. Environmental Protection Agency, Washington, DC. May 2003 [online]. Available: http://oaspub. epa.gov/eims/eimscomm.getfile?p_download_id=36941 [accessed June 10, 2008].

EPA (U.S. Environmental Protection Agency). 2003c. The Feasibility of Performing Cumulative Risk Assessments for Mixtures of Disinfection By-Products in Drinking Water. EPA/600/R-03/051. National Center for Environmental Assessment, U.S. Environmental Protection Agency, Cincinnati, OH. June 2003 [online]. Available: http://cfpub.epa.gov/ncea/cfm/recordisplay.cfm?deid=56834 [accessed July 22, 2008].

EPA (U.S. Environmental Protection Agency). 2005a. Guidelines for Carcinogen Risk Assessment. EPA/630/P-03/001F. Risk Assessment Forum, U.S. Environmental Protection Agency, Washington, DC. March 2005 [online]. Available: http://cfpub. epa.gov/ncea/cfm/recordisplay.cfm?deid=116283 [accessed Sept. 2, 2008].

EPA (U.S. Environmental Protection Agency). 2005b. Supplemental Guidance for Assessing Susceptibility from Early-Life Exposure to Carcinogens. EPA/630/R-03/03F. Risk Assessment Forum, U.S. Environmental Protection Agency, Washington, DC. March 2005 [online]. Available: http://www.epa.gov/iris/children 032505.pdf [accessed June 16, 2008).

EPA (U.S. Environmental Protection Agency). 2006. 1996 National Air Toxics Assessment Exposure and Risk Data. Technology Transfer Network National Air Toxics Assessment, U.S. Environmental Protection Agency [online]. Available: http:// www.epa.gov/ttn/atw/nata/ted/exporisk.html [accessed July 22, 2008].

EPA (U.S. Environmental Protection Agency). 2007a. 1,1,1-Trichloroethane (CASRN 71-55-6). Integrated Risk Information System, U.S. Environmental Protection Agency [online]. Available: http://www.epa.gov/ncea/iris/subst/0197.htm [accessed July 23, 2008].

EPA (U.S. Environmental Protection Agency). 2007b. Provisional Peer Reviewed Toxicity Values for Dimethyl Phthalate (CASRN 131-11-3). Superfund Health Risk Technical Support Center, National Center for Environmental Assessment, Office of Research and Development, U.S. Environmental Protection Agency, Cincinnati, OH. September 25, 2007.

EPA (U.S. Environmental Protection Agency). 2007c. Risk Management Decisions for Individual N-methyl Carbamate Pesticides. Pesticides, U.S. Environmental Protection Agency [online]. Available: http://www.epa.gov/pesticides/cumulative/ carbamate_risk_mgmt.htm [accessed July 22, 2008].

EPA (U.S. Environmental Protection Agency). 2007d. 1996 National-Scale Air Toxics Assessment. Overview: EPA's Use of Results. Technology Transfer Network, U.S.

Environmental Protection Agency [online]. Available: http://www.epa.gov/ttn/
    atw/nata/ur.html [accessed July 22, 2008].
EPA (U.S. Environmental Protection Agency). 2007e. 1996 National-Scale Air Toxics
    Assessment. Background on Risk Characterization. Technology Transfer Network,
    U.S. Environmental Protection Agency [online]. Available: http://www.epa.gov/
    ttn/atw/nata/riskbg.html [accessed July 22, 2008].
EPA (U.S. Environmental Protection Agency). 2007f. 1996 National-Scale Air Toxics
    Assessment. Summary of Results. Technology Transfer Network, U.S. Environ-
    mental Protection Agency [online]. Available: http://www.epa.gov/ttn/atw/
    nata/risksum.html [accessed July 22, 2008].
EPA (U.S. Environmental Protection Agency). 2007g. Concepts, Methods, and Data
    Sources for Cumulative Health Risk Assessment of Multiple Chemicals, Expo-
    sures and Effects: A Resource Document. EPA/600/R-06/013F. National Center
    for Environmental Assessment, Office of Research and Development, U.S. Envi-
    ronmental Protection Agency, Cincinnati, OH, in collaboration with U.S. Depart-
    ment of Energy, Argonne National Laboratory, Environmental Assessment Divi-
    sion, Argonne, IL. August 2007 [online]. Available: http://cfpub.epa.gov/ncea/
    cfm/recordisplay.cfm?deid=190187 [accessed Nov. 12, 2008].
EPA (U.S. Environmental Protection Agency). 2008a. Target Compounds and Analytes.
    Superfund Analytical Services/Contact Laboratory Program, U.S. Environmental
    Protection Agency [online]. Available: http://www.epa.gov/superfund/programs/
    clp/target.htm [accessed July 23, 2008].
EPA (U.S. Environmental Protection Agency). 2008b. IRIS Glossary. Integrated Risk
    Information System (IRIS), U.S. Environmental Protection Agency [online].
    Available: http://www.epa.gov/ncea/iris/help_gloss.htm#r [accessed July 23,
    2008].
EPA (U.S. Environmental Protection Agency). 2008c. EPA's Integrated Risk Information
    System: Assessment Development Procedures. IRIS Process (2008 Update). Na-
    tional Center for Environmental Assessment, U.S. Environmental Protection
    Agency. April 2008 [online]. Available: http://cfpub.epa.gov/ncea/cfm/record
    isplay.cfm?deid=190045 [accessed June 11, 2008].
EPA (U.S. Environmental Protection Agency). 2008d. Assessing Pesticide Cumulative
    Risk. Pesticides, U.S. Environmental Protection Agency [online]. Available:
    http://www.epa.gov/pesticides/cumulative/index.htm [accessed July 22, 2008].
EPA (U.S. Environmental Protection Agency). 2008e. Common Mechanism Groups;
    Cumulative Exposure and Risk Assessment. Pesticides, U.S. Environmental Pro-
    tection Agency [online]. Available: http://www.epa.gov/pesticides/cumulative/
    common_mech_groups.htm [accessed July 22, 2008].
EPA (U.S. Environmental Protection Agency). 2008f. Proposed Approach for Estimation
    of Bin-Specific Cancer Potency Factors for Inhalation Exposure to Asbestos. Of-
    fice of Solid Waste and Emergency Response, U.S. Environmental Protection
    Agency [online]. Available: http://www.epa.gov/oswer/riskassessment/asbestos/
    pdfs/2008_prop_asbestos_approach.pdf [accessed July 22, 2008].
EPA (U.S. Environmental Protection Agency). 2008g. Revised N-Methyl Carbamate
    Cumulative Risk Assessment. Office of Pesticide Programs, U.S. Environmental
    Protection Agency [online]. Available: http://www.epa.gov/pesticides/cumulative/
    common_mech_groups.htm#carbamate [accessed July 22, 2008].
Gustafson, J.B., J.G. Tell, and D. Orem. 1997. Selection of Representative TPH fractions
    Based on Fate and Transport Considerations. Total Petroleum Hydrocarbon Crite-
    ria Working Group Series, Vol. 3. Amherst, MA: Amherst Scientific Publishers

[online]. Available: http://www.aehs.com/publications/catalog/contents/Volume3. pdf [accessed July 23, 2008].

ILSI (International Life Science Institute). 1999. A Framework for Cumulative Risk Assessment, B. Mileson, E. Faustman, S. Olin, P. B. Ryan, S. Ferenc, and T. Burke, eds. Washington, DC: International Life Science Institute [online]. Available: http://rsi.ilsi.org/NR/rdonlyres/613A82AA-E74F-40B2-BA38-1548A9C6AD8C/0/rsiframrpt.pdf [accessed July 23, 2008].

MADEP (Massachusetts Department of Environmental Protection). 2002. Characterization of Risks Posed by Petroleum Contaminated Sites: Implementation of MADEP VPH/EPH Approach. Final October 31, 2002. Policy No. WSC-02-411. Commonwealth of Massachusetts Executive Office of Environmental Affairs, Department of Environmental Protection [online]. Available: http://www.mass.gov/dep/cleanup/laws/02-411.pdf [accessed July 22, 2008].

MADEP (Massachusetts Department of Environmental Protection). 2003. Updated Petroleum Hydrocarbon Fraction Toxicity Values for the VPH/EPH/APH Methodology. Office of Research and Standards, Massachusetts Department of Environmental Protection, Boston, MA. November 2003 [online]. Available: http://www.mass.gov/dep/cleanup/laws/tphtox03.pdf [accessed July 22, 2008].

Norberg, L., and G. Wahlström. 1988. Anaesthetic effects of flurazepam alone and in combination with thiopental or hexobarbital evaluated with an EEG-threshold method in male rats. Arch. int. Pharmacodyn. 292:45-57.

OEHHA (Office of Environmental Health Hazard Assessment). 2008. Toxicity Criteria Database. Office of Environmental Health Hazard Assessment, California Environmental Protection Agency [online]. Available: http://www.oehha.ca.gov/risk/chemicalDB//index.asp [accessed July 23, 2008].

Teuschler, L.K., G.E. Rice, C.R. Wilkes, J.C. Lipscomb, and F.W. Power. 2004. A feasibility study of cumulative risk assessment methods for drinking water disinfection by-product mixtures. J. Toxicol. Environ. Health Part A 67(8-10):755-777.

Van den Berg, M., L. Birnbaum, A.T. Bosveld, B. Brunström, P. Cook, M. Feeley, J.P. Giesy, A. Hanberg, R. Hasegawa, S.W. Kennedy, T. Kubiak, J.C. Larsen, F.X. van Leeuwen, A.K. Liem, C. Nolt, R.E. Peterson, L. Poellinger, S. Safe, D. Schrenk, D. Tillitt, M. Tysklind, M. Younes, F. Waern, and T. Zacharewski. 1998. Toxic equivalency factors (TEFs) for PCBs, PCDDs, PCDFs for humans and wildlife. Environ. Health Perspect. 106(12):775-792.

Van den Berg, M., L.S. Birnbaum, M. Denison, M. De Vito, W. Farland, M. Feeley, H. Fiedler, H. Hakansson, A. Hanberg, L. Haws, M. Rose, S. Safe, D. Schrenk, C. Tohyama, A. Tritscher, J. Tuomisto, M. Tysklind, N. Walker, and R.E. Peterson. 2006. The 2005 World Health Organization reevaluation of human and mammalian toxic equivalency factors for dioxins and dioxin-like compounds. Toxicol. Sci. 93(2):223-241.

5

Cumulative Risk Assessment of Phthalates and Related Chemicals

Our understanding of the toxicity of phthalates and the associated underlying mechanisms has improved considerably in the last few years. Effects on reproductive development in the male constitute one of the most sensitive end points. Some phthalates—such as DBP, BBP, DEHP, and DINP—are able to disrupt male sexual differentiation by interfering with androgen biosynthesis; this culminates in what has been described as the phthalate syndrome or more generally as the androgen-insufficiency syndrome. Because the chemicals have a similar effect spectrum, it is likely that they act in concert when they occur together. However, not only phthalates can disrupt male sexual differentiation. As discussed in Chapter 3, other classes of chemicals, so-called antiandrogens, are also able to interfere with male development by opposing the actions of fetal androgens in different ways. Antiandrogens can block the effects of fetal androgens by antagonizing the androgen receptor (AR) or can reduce concentrations of fetal androgens by inhibiting key enzymes responsible for the conversion of precursor steroids into androgens. Other chemicals exhibit mixed mechanisms, for example, by both inhibiting enzymes and blocking the AR. Thus, there may be considerable potential for cumulative effects of phthalates and other classes of antiandrogens in that any interference with AR-related effects may result in components of the phthalate syndrome.

This chapter assesses the empirical evidence of combined effects of several phthalates, of nonphthalate antiandrogens, and of phthalates and these other antiandrogens. Because of the importance of developmental effects, the overview focuses almost exclusively on experimental evidence from reproductive-toxicity studies. Many published experimental mixture studies were motivated by an interest in determining the type of combination effect (for example, additive or synergistic) of the agents involved. That effort often required the administration of doses of test chemicals that were associated with measurable effects but were far removed from exposures experienced by humans. What will lend further urgency to calls to conduct cumulative risk assessment is the demonstration of combined effects at low doses of each mixture component. For that reason, the committee scrutinized the evidence in the literature particularly with respect to low-dose combined effects.

After examining the empirical evidence, this chapter considers options for conducting cumulative risk assessment of phthalates and other antiandrogens. First, several questions are addressed to set the stage for considering various approaches. Which phthalates should be subjected to cumulative risk assessment? Should other antiandrogens be included? If so, which ones? What criteria should be used to group phthalates and other antiandrogens for cumulative risk assessment? Next, approaches to quantitative assessments of cumulative effects are discussed. For cumulative risk assessments of dioxins and other chemical classes, the toxicity equivalency (TEQ) concept has gained broad acceptance and is in widespread use. Accordingly, this chapter addresses whether the TEQ concept presents a practicable option for cumulative risk assessment of phthalates and other antiandrogens or whether alternative approaches should be adopted. The chapter concludes with a discussion of possible stepped approaches to cumulative risk assessment of phthalates and other antiandrogens.

CRITERIA FOR CHOOSING DOSE ADDITION OR INDEPENDENT ACTION AS A DEFAULT EVALUATION METHOD

Dose addition and *independent action* (here used synonymously with *response addition*) provide two possible approaches to dealing with the mixture issue. However, when one is faced with the task of evaluating specific mixtures, the issue arises as to whether either of the two concepts is appropriate for the mixture in question and should be chosen for assessment. That question becomes all the more important when the two concepts produce different predictions of mixture effects. However, in only a few cases have dose addition and independent action been evaluated together against the same set of experimental mixture data with the aim of establishing whether either approach produces valid predictions of combined effects (for a review, see Kortenkamp et al. 2007). As pointed out by the U.S. Environmental Protection Agency (EPA 2000), the empirical basis of choosing between dose addition and independent action as a default approach for risk assessment is not strong. The decision in favor of either approach as a default for mixture risk assessment is based largely on perceptions of whether the scientific assumptions that underpin dose addition or independent action are met. For such purposes, the two concepts have been allied to broad mechanisms of combined toxicity, as described below.

Dose addition is often stated to be applicable to mixtures composed of chemicals that have a similar or common mechanism of action (EPA 1986, 2000, 2002; COT 2002). However, the original paper by Loewe and Muischneck (1926) contains little that roots dose addition in mechanistic considerations; the idea of similar action probably derives from the "dilution" principle, which forms the basis of this approach. Because chemicals are viewed as dilutions of each other, it may be implicitly assumed that they must act via common or similar mechanisms.

In contrast, independent action is widely assumed to be appropriate for mixtures of agents that have diverse or dissimilar mechanisms of action. Although it is rarely stated, that assumption probably stems from the stochastic principles that guided the development of the approach. Acting independently is equated with the notion of acting through different mechanisms. By activating differing effector chains, the argument goes, every component of a mixture of dissimilarly acting chemicals provokes effects independently of all other agents that are present, and this feature appears to lend itself to statistical concepts of independent events. Independent action is often held to be the default assessment concept when the similarity criteria of dose addition appear to be violated (COT 2002). If "dissimilar action" is taken implicitly as the simple negation of "similar action," it is then assumed that independent action must hold (with the further implicit assumption that only two choices are available), even without further proof that the underlying mechanisms satisfy the dissimilarity criterion.

Although those ideas are plausible, their application to specific combinations of chemicals is far from clear-cut. One major difficulty lies in defining reliable criteria for similarity of mechanisms of action. Often, the induction of the same phenomenologic effect is deemed sufficient for accepting similarity of action. However, that could be inappropriate for some combinations of chemicals that operate by distinct molecular mechanisms. At the other extreme of the spectrum of opinion, the similarity assumption might require an identical molecular mechanism involving the same active intermediates. That position, with its strict similarity criterion, may mean that few chemicals qualify for inclusion in mixture-effects assessments and many others that provoke the same response are left out. In effect, that approach would provide an unrealistically narrow perspective on existing mixtures. A middle position is occupied by the view that interactions with the same site, tissue, or target organ should qualify for similarity (EPA 1986, 1989; Mileson et al. 1998).

SIMILAR OR DISSIMILAR ACTION: A DEFAULT CONCEPT FOR CUMULATIVE RISK ASSESSMENT OF PHTHALATES AND OTHER ANTIANDROGENS?

It is not immediately obvious which criteria should be used to classify phthalates as similarly or dissimilarly acting chemicals. EPA (2000) has recommended that decisions about whether to use dose addition or independent action should be based on information about the toxic and physiologic processes involved, the single-chemical dose-response relationships, and the type of response data available. If information about target tissue concentrations is available, such judgments can focus on the toxic mechanism of action within that tissue. With phthalates, external doses, but not target-tissue doses have been used, and in such cases EPA (2000) demands that decisions about similarity of action consider all processes, including uptake, metabolism, elimination, and toxic mechanism.

Although there is little detail about the precise uptake mechanisms of phthalates, it is clear that they all undergo hydrolysis to produce phthalate monoesters that are then transported to their site of action. In the case of many monoesters, there is a rapid reduction in fetal testosterone production in the Leydig cells of the testes and a consequent indirect effect through down-regulation of key enzymes important in the transport and conversion of steroid precursors. The resulting impairment of Leydig cell function triggers a decrease in androgen-mediated gene expression. Because androgen action is a key driver in sexual differentiation, disturbance of androgen-mediated development gives rise to profound effects on the male reproductive system (Foster 2005). Phthalates can be judged to exhibit a similar mechanism of action, with dose addition the appropriate default assessment approach according to EPA guidelines. However, differences in phthalate metabolism may lead to dissimilarities in the precise toxic mechanism. For example, some metabolites of DEHP (MEOHP and MEHHP) can antagonize the AR (Stroheker et al. 2005), but that is not the case for all metabolites of phthalates. Furthermore, some phthalates can induce some peroxisome-proliferator-activated receptor isoforms, but others lack this ability (Bility et al. 2004). Should the mechanisms of action of those phthalates therefore be judged to be dissimilar and independent action adopted according to other suggestions in EPA guidelines?

EPA (2000) also stipulated that to qualify for dose addition, all dose-response curves should be congruent. That requirement is not met by phthalates. Dose-response studies have revealed a large variety of shapes (Rider et al. 2008; Howdeshell et al. 2008). Does that mean that the concept of dose addition should not be used in connection with phthalate mixtures?

The demand for congruent curves may be derived from a misunderstanding of the mathematical features of the dilution principle that underpins dose addition. It appears to have been thought that the principle requires a constant proportionality between the doses of chemicals in a mixture that produce a given effect. For chemicals with different potency, a chemical may have to be administered at a dose that is a multiple of another chemical's dose to achieve the same effect of a specific size. Although that proposition would lead to dose addition, it does not follow that the dose-response curves of all dose-additive mixture components have to be congruent. Congruent curves result only if it is also demanded that the multiple is constant for all effect levels. For example, let 10 dose units of substance A induce an effect of 12 (on an arbitrary scale), and assume that only 5 dose units of substance B are required to produce the same effect. In that case, there is a proportionality factor of 2 between the doses of the two chemicals. Congruent shapes of the dose-response curves result if the same proportionality of 2 is preserved at all other effect levels. Thus, in this arbitrary example, 20 dose units of A and 10 dose units of B each would produce the same but larger effect of, say, 17. Now consider mixture effects under the principle of dose addition. Accordingly, 5 dose units of A and 2.5 of B are expected to produce an effect of 12. To provoke an effect of 17, dose addition would re-quire application of 10 dose units of A and 5 of B. However, dose addition would apply even if the demand of constant proportionality between the effect doses of the two chemicals is not fulfilled. For example, let 20 dose units of A produce an effect of 17, as before, but assume that B has a lower potency at this effect level, such that 16 dose units are necessary to yield an effect of 17. Dose addition would still be applicable: it can be predicted that 10 units of A and 8 units of B combined should produce an effect of 17. Thus, although the addi-tional requirement of constant proportionality is a precondition for the applica-tion of relative potencies and toxicity equivalence factors (TEFs), it is not neces-sary for the general use of dose addition, which also works with curves of different shapes (Berenbaum 1989; Hass et al. 2007; Howdeshell et al. 2008). Moreover, the existence of congruent dose-response curves for mixture compo-nents does not constitute evidence for or against dose additivity. Given the above discussion, EPA may wish to revise some of its guidance (for example, EPA 2000).

The application of the criteria used by EPA (2000) for making choices be-tween dose addition and independent action for phthalate mixtures leaves ambi-guities that cannot readily be resolved without further empirical evidence, which would overrule any such heuristic arguments in any case.

The committee concludes that the criteria applied by EPA are too narrow and restrictive because they leave out other chemicals that can disrupt male sex-ual differentiation but in ways that differ in some respects from phthalates (see Chapter 3). With phthalates and other antiandrogens, the case can be made for adopting a physiologic approach to analyzing toxic mechanisms of action with respect to similarity or dissimilarity. If it is recognized that the driver of male sexual differentiation during development is the effect of androgen action, it may be irrelevant whether the hormones' effects are disrupted by interference with steroid synthesis, by antagonism of the AR, or by some other mechanism (for example, affecting consequences of AR activation). The resulting biologic effects with all their consequences for male sexual differentiation may be simi-lar, although the molecular details of toxic mechanisms—including metabolism, distribution and elimination—may differ profoundly in many respects. Judged from such a perspective, a focus on phthalates to the exclusion of other antian-drogens (or other more esoterically acting agents) not only would be artificial but could imply serious underestimation of cumulative risks posed by agents to which there is coexposure.

In contrast, the differences in the mechanisms of action of phthalates and other antiandrogens could mean that the independent-action principle is better suited for evaluating the combined effects of chemicals. That issue cannot be decided without considering empirical evidence. Accordingly, the question be-comes, are there data in the recent literature that can help to resolve some of these difficulties?

EXPERIMENTAL EVIDENCE OF CUMULATIVE EFFECTS OF COMBINATIONS OF PHTHALATES AND OTHER ANTIANDROGENS

This section reviews experimental studies of combined effects of several phthalates, of other antiandrogens, and of phthalates and other antiandrogens. Rather than a comprehensive review of the literature, the primary aim is to examine empirical evidence of combined effects of phthalates and other antiandrogens. A secondary aim is to assess whether experimentally observed mixture effects agree quantitatively with the additivity expectations derived from dose addition. In dealing with those issues, it is important to recognize that dose addition and independent action often yield identical, experimentally indistinguishable, or trivially distinct predictions of additive combined effects. However, under some circumstances, the two concepts produce additivity predictions that differ enough to be distinguished experimentally. It is then possible to discern which concept better agrees with observed effects. In such cases, the argument for using the better predictor (dose addition or independent action) as an approximation for mixture risk assessment is strong. For that reason, published data will, wherever possible, be examined in relation to agreement with dose addition or independent action.

It is not always straightforward to judge the quality of agreement between experimentally observed data and predictions based on dose addition or independent action. Although it is frequently possible to distinguish qualitatively which of the two concepts approximates the data better, there are no generally accepted criteria for statistical assessments. One approach is to demand that the predictions overlap with the confidence intervals of the experimental data, but this may lead to an overly strict criteria for agreement. An alternative would be to consider how variations in single-chemical response data affect the uncertainties associated with predictions by using boot-strapping methods. In that way, confidence intervals for predictions can be calculated (Hass et al. 2007). The agreement with observations can then be judged statistically by considering the overlap between the confidence intervals of the prediction with that of the experimental data. Frequently, however, data quality and experimental design (or the lack of information presented in the literature) do not allow the use of such approaches. In the absence of generally accepted criteria for assessing agreement with predicted additivity, qualitative judgments often have to be made without the use of statistical reasoning. Although that approach may be unsatisfactory, the committee emphasizes that there are currently no practical alternatives, owing to a lack of theoretical foundations able to underpin better practice.

Combinations of Phthalates Yield Good Evidence of Dose-Additive Effects

Howdeshell et al. (2007) examined a binary mixture of DBP and DEHP. Those two phthalates are thought to have a common mechanism of action, but they yield different metabolites. Pregnant Sprague-Dawley rats (six dams per dose) were exposed to the phthalates during gestation days 14-18 at 500 mg/kg-d each, both singly and in combination. Their male offspring were examined for a wide array of effects typical of disruption of male sexual differentiation, including changes in fetal testosterone production, changes in anogenital distance, epididymal agenesis, retained nipples, gubernacular agenesis, hypospadias, and number of animals with malformations. Dose addition generally predicted larger effects than independent action, although for some end points the two concepts predicted equal effects. It is not possible to duplicate the dose-addition predictions given by the authors, because they were based on unpublished dose-response data on the individual phthalates. However, the authors observed that the responses generally agreed well with dose addition and were higher than the additivity expectations derived from independent action for changes in anogenital distance, epididymal agenesis, and number of malformed males. The study indicates that dose addition provides fairly good predictions of many of the effects that make up the androgen-insufficiency syndrome. Independent action often underestimated the observed responses.

Recently, Howdeshell et al. (2008) presented the results of a mixture study of five phthalates in which suppression of fetal testosterone production at gestation day 18 was measured as a result of exposure of pregnant Sprague-Dawley rats. BBP, DBP, DEHP, DIBP, and DPP were combined in a fixed ratio. The committee's reanalysis of the raw data revealed that for testosterone reduction, dose-addition and independent-action predictions were generally similar (see Figure 5-1 and Appendix C for further details and analysis). Over a large range of effect levels, the observed reductions in testosterone production agreed well with the responses predicted by either model, although there were small, statistically significant differences between the dose-addition prediction and the observed data.

Combinations of Antiandrogens Follow the Principle of Dose Addition

By using the isobole method (an application of dose addition), Nellemann et al. (2003) found that the fungicides procymidone and vinclozolin, both AR antagonists, additively inhibited testosterone binding to the AR. Administration of a 1:1 mixture to castrated, testosterone-treated male rats led to dose-additive alterations in reproductive organ weights, androgen concentrations, and AR-dependent gene expression. Birkhoj et al. (2004) extended the use of the isobole method to three-component mixtures of the pesticides deltamethrin, methiocarb, and prochloraz. An equimolar mixture of the three additively suppressed AR activation in vitro. When a combination of those three with simazin and tribenuron-methyl was given to castrated testosterone-treated rats, changes in adrenal gland and levator ani weights and in expression of AR-associated genes were observed. The combination of all five chemicals had effects that were not found for the individual pesticides, but whether the effects were dose-additive could not be assessed by the authors.

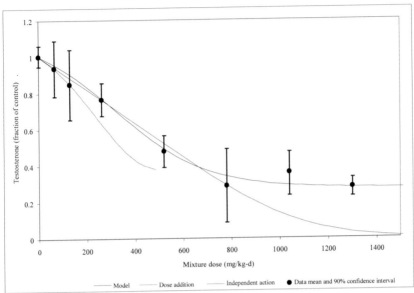

FIGURE 5-1 The committee's reanalysis of the combined effects of five phthalates on suppression of testosterone production (Howdeshell et al. 2008). See Appendix C for further details.

A mixture of the AR antagonists procymidone and vinclozolin was evaluated in the Hershberger assay (reviewed by Gray et al. 2001). Although it was not possible to evaluate the dose-additivity prediction with the information provided, the mixture appeared to exhibit effect addition in percentage reduction of ventral prostate and levator ani weights.[1]

Hass et al. (2007) examined a mixture of three AR antagonists (vinclozolin, flutamide, and procymidone) in an extended developmental-toxicity model in the rat. Disruption of sexual differentiation in male offspring was studied; the end points were changes in anogenital distance (AGD) and nipple retention (NR). On the basis of AGD changes, the joint effect of the three chemicals was predicted well by dose addition, but the observed effects on NR were slightly greater than those predicted by dose addition. In this study, the agreement between dose addition and experimentally observed responses was evaluated statistically by using boot-strapping methods.

Metzdorff et al. (2007) analyzed further the material from the Hass et al. (2007) study by following effects typical of antiandrogen action through different levels of biologic complexity. Changes in reproductive organ weights and of androgen-regulated gene expression in prostates of male rat pups were chosen as

---

[1]In effect addition, the combined effect of several chemicals is calculated by summing the responses to the individual agents at the doses present in the mixture.

end points for extensive dose-response studies. With all the end points, the joint effects of the three antiandrogens were dose-additive. That conclusion is supported by a statistical evaluation of the agreement between dose-addition predictions and observations that the study authors conducted by judging overlap of confidence intervals of the prediction and the experimental data.

In the examples presented here, the AR antagonists evaluated in the studies are known to induce antiandrogenicity by the same mechanism.

Combinations of Phthalates with Other Antiandrogens Also Exhibit Dose-Additive Effects

Hotchkiss et al. (2004) investigated a mixture of BBP and linuron, an antiandrogen capable of antagonizing the AR and disrupting steroid synthesis. The combination decreased testosterone production and caused alterations in androgen-organized tissues and malformations of external genitalia. Quantitative additivity expectations based on the effects of the single chemicals were not calculated in this study, so agreement with dose addition or independent action cannot be assessed. However, the combination of BBP and linuron always produced greater effects than each chemical on its own. That result demonstrates that BBP and linuron can act together to produce an effect spectrum typical of disruption of androgen action.

Rider et al. (2008) conducted mixture experiments with the three phthalates BBP, DBP, and DEHP in combination with the antiandrogens vinclozolin, procymidone, linuron, and prochloraz. The mixture was given to pregnant rats with the aim of examining the male offspring for a variety of developmental effects typical of antiandrogens. Its components have a variety of antiandrogenic mechanisms of action. Vinclozolin and procymidone are AR antagonists, and linuron and prochloraz exhibit a mixed mechanism of action: inhibiting steroid synthesis and blocking the steroid receptor. In calculating additivity expectations, the authors used historical data from their laboratory; however, the studies sometimes had dosing regimens that differed from those used in the mixture experiments. Data on the effects of some individual phthalates were not available. To bridge that data gap for the purpose of computing additivity expectations, it was assumed that the three phthalates were equipotent. Despite some uncertainty inevitably introduced by that assumption, dose addition gave predictions of combined effects of the mixed-mode antiandrogens that agreed better with the observed responses than did the expectations derived from independent action. For a number of end points—including seminal vesicle weights, epididymal agenesis, and NR—there was reasonable agreement with dose addition. For others, such as hypospadias, the observed effects exceeded the dose-addition expectation. A statistical evaluation of the agreement between dose addition and experimental data was not provided by the study authors, and the committee judged that such an analysis was not possible on the basis of the published data.

Nevertheless, independent action led to considerable underestimation of the observed combined effects in all cases.

Table 5-1 summarizes the mixture studies that allowed quantitative comparison of observed combined effects with predictions derived from dose addition. The committee notes that the studies revealed a large variety of differently shaped dose-response curves for phthalates acting individually (Howdeshell et al. 2008; Rider et al. 2008) and antiandrogens acting individually (Hass et al. 2007). The studies provide empirical examples in which chemicals with similar mechanisms can have entirely different dose-response curves.

COMBINED EFFECTS OF LOW DOSES OF PHTHALATES AND OTHER ANTIANDROGENS

When it comes to judging the risks associated with low-level exposures, there are marked differences between the chemical-by-chemical approach to risk assessment and evaluations that take mixture effects into account. Where single-chemical risk assessments might yield the verdict "absence of risk," dose addition or independent action might yield the opposite conclusion.

An obvious deduction from the dilution principle of dose addition is the expectation that every component at any dose contributes, in proportion to its prevalence, to the overall mixture toxicity. Whether the individual doses of mixture components are effective on their own does not matter.

The idea can be illustrated by considering a dose-fractionation experiment (see Figure 5-2), where a dose of 4×10^{-2} arbitrary dose units produces an effect of measurable magnitude. The same effect will be obtained when the chemical is administered in 10 simultaneous portions of 4×10^{-3} dose units, even though the response to each one of those dose fractions is not measurable (or is exactly zero if there is a true dose threshold). If dose addition applies, the same holds when 10 portions of 10 chemicals with identical response curves are used. Thus, combined effects should also result from chemicals at doses associated with zero effect (dose thresholds) or even lower doses, provided that sufficiently large numbers of components sum to a suitably high effect dose.

Theoretically, the situation described above is not necessarily the case ith independent action where simultaneous exposure to large numbers of chemicals at doses associated with zero effects is expected to produce a zero mixture effect. An experimental assessment of that idea, however, is complicated by the fact that true zero effect levels (dose thresholds), if they exist at doses larger than zero, are difficult to determine empirically. Particularly in the case of mixtures of a large number of components, that proposition forces clear distinctions between zero effects and small, albeit statistically insignificant effects. For example, under independent action the combined effect of 100 chemicals, each of which individually provokes a response of 1%, will be 63% of a maximally inducible effect. If each of the 100 chemicals produces an effect of only 0.1%,

TABLE 5-1 Mixture Studies of Phthalates and Other Antiandrogens

End Point	Assay or Organism	Mixture Components	Assessment	Reference
Mixtures of phthalates				
In vivo, suppression of testosterone synthesis	Sprague-Dawley rats exposed in utero	BBP, DBP, DEHP, DINP, DPP	~ DA or IA[a]	Howdeshell et al. 2008
Mixtures of antiandrogens				
In vitro, inhibition of androgen-induced AR activation	AR CHO cell-based AR reporter gene assay	Procymidone, vinclozolin	= DA	Nellemann et al. 2003
In vitro, inhibition of androgen-induced AR activation	CHO cell-based AR reporter gene assay (modified)	Deltamethrin methiocarb, prochloraz, 2 inactive substances	= DA	Birkhoj et al. 2004
In vivo, changes in AR-dependent gene expression	Castrated testosterone-treated male Wistar rats (extended Hershberger assay)	Procymidone, vinclozolin	= DA	Nellemann et al. 2003
In vivo, changes in hormone concentrations: LH and FSH	Castrated testosterone-treated male Wistar rats (extended Hershberger assay)	Procymidone, vinclozolin	= DA	Nellemann et al. 2003
In vivo, changes in reproductive organ weights	Castrated testosterone-treated male Wistar rats (extended Hershberger assay)	Procymidone, vinclozolin	= DA	Nellemann et al. 2003
In vivo, effects on androgen-regulated gene expression in prostate	Male Wistar rats exposed in utero and postnatally	Vinclozolin, flutamide, procymidone	= DA	Metzdorff et al. 2007
In vivo, changes in reproductive organ weights	Male Wistar rats exposed in utero and postnatally	Vinclozolin, flutamide, procymidone	= DA	Metzdorff et al. 2007
In vivo, changes in AGD	Male Wistar rats exposed in utero and postnatally	Vinclozolin, flutamide, procymidone	= DA	Hass et al. 2007
In vivo, NR	Male Wistar rats exposed in utero and postnatally	Vinclozolin, flutamide, procymidone	= DA at low effective doses; > DA in median effects range[b]	Hass et al. 2007

TABLE 5-1 Continued

End Point	Assay or Organism	Mixture Components	Assessment	Reference
Mixtures of phthalates and antiandrogens				
In vivo, changes in AGD	Male Sprague-Dawley rats exposed in utero	Vinclozolin, prochloraz, procymidone, linuron, BBP, DBP, DEHP	~ DA	Rider et al. 2008
In vivo, changes in NR	Male Sprague-Dawley rats exposed in utero	Vinclozolin, prochloraz, procymidone, linuron, BBP, DBP, DEHP	~ DA	Rider et al. 2008
In vivo, changes in seminal vesicle weights	Male Sprague-Dawley rats exposed in utero	Vinclozolin, prochloraz, procymidone, linuron, BBP, DBP, DEHP	= DA	Rider et al. 2008
In vivo, hypospadias	Male Sprague-Dawley rats exposed in utero	Vinclozolin, prochloraz, procymidone, linuron, BBP, DBP, DEHP	> DA	Rider et al. 2008

Note: AR, androgen receptor; CHO, Chinese hamster ovary; DA, dose addition; EDx, effective dose at x response level; FSH, follicle-stimulating hormone; IA, independent action; LH, luteinizing hormone; NR, nipple retention.
[a]EDx observed / EDx predicted ≈ 1/0.9.
[b]EDx observed / EDx predicted ≈ 1/1.7.

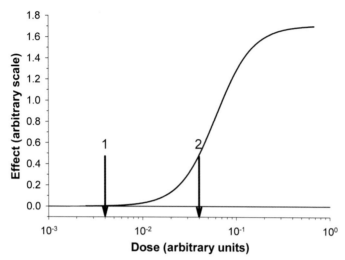

FIGURE 5-2 Illustration of a "sham" mixture experiment with chemicals that all exhibit the same dose-response curve. At the low dose to the left (arrow 1, 4×10^{-3} dose units), the effect is hardly observable. A combination of 10 agents at that dose (arrow 2, total dose, 4×10^{-2} dose units) produces a significant combined effect, consistent with expectations based on dose addition.

the expected combined effect will be 9.5%. With the test systems used in toxicology, distinguishing such small effects from those seen in untreated controls is practically impossible.

It is well established that regulatory toxicology has dealt with the problem of small responses at low doses by using uncertainty factors to approximate zero effect levels for the purpose of estimating "safe" exposures of humans. As a starting point for establishing such "allowable," "acceptable," or "tolerable" exposures, no-observed-adverse-effect levels (NOAELs) are used. The NOAEL is the highest dose or exposure at which no statistically or biologically adverse effects can be identified (EPA 1994). It is used as a point of departure for estimating tolerable human exposures by dividing by uncertainty factors.

A number of shortcomings of NOAELs, however, have been identified. There are problems with a single numerical value adequately reflecting study size and the shape of the underlying dose-response curves (Crump 1984; Slob 1999). NOAELs are not fixed attributes of toxic substances; rather, they reflect features of experimental design. Larger experimental studies will detect effects at lower exposures and thus will yield lower NOAELs (Crump 2002; Scholze and Kortenkamp 2007).

To deal with those conceptual problems, the benchmark dose (BMD) has been developed as a statistical tool to determine acceptable exposures to a chemical (Crump 1984). The BMD is a dose that causes a prescribed effect (generally within or close to the experimentally observed range) and is estimated by fitting a regression model to experimental data. Compared with NOAELs, BMDs have the advantage of yielding lower numerical values with data of poor quality. Numerous papers have evaluated the properties of BMDs (summarized in Crump 2002), and the topic has been the subject of a National Research Council evaluation (NRC 2000). Accordingly, the committee felt that an in-depth discussion of the threshold problem in toxicology and the issues surrounding the use of NOAELs and BMDs as the basis of toxicologic risk assessment was outside the scope of this report. It suffices to say that BMDs have been endorsed by EPA as an acceptable replacement of NOAELs whenever appropriate quantitative data are available (EPA 1994). That conclusion is supported by an evaluation of a large database of developmental-toxicity experiments to compare BMD approaches with NOAELs. For continuous response variables, BMDs associated with 5% additional risk produced dose estimates similar to NOAELs (Allen et al. 1994).

The issue to be examined here is whether there is evidence that phthalates, in combination with other phthalates or with other antiandrogens, exhibit combined effects at doses that are used in risk assessment by regulatory agencies worldwide as points of departure (PODs) for estimating tolerable exposures of humans. Those PODs are typically NOAELs or lower confidence limits of BMDs (BMDLs). A complicating factor is that the majority of combined-effect studies with the chemicals were not carried out with the intention of addressing the low-dose-mixture issue directly. That gap can be bridged by reanalyzing published papers, but the task requires considerations of methodologic issues related to the concept and design of low-dose-mixture studies.

Mixture Studies with Doses around Points of Departure for Risk Assessment: Methodologic Considerations

A requirement for experimental studies intended to address the issue of mixture effects at doses around PODs for regulatory risk assessment is that such estimates are derived for each mixture component by using the same assay system (and end point) as chosen for the mixture study, ideally under identical experimental conditions. Ignoring that demand can lead to the inadvertent administration of some or all mixture components at doses exceeding their PODs, which would undermine the aim of the experiment. But delivery of doses smaller than PODs, either by design or by accident, might present problems if the experimental system lacks the statistical power to detect small effects. For example, it would be futile to attempt an experiment in which two agents are combined at one hundredth of their individual PODs. The resulting mixture effect, if it exists, would be too small to be detectable in most cases, and the experiment would be inconclusive.

Accordingly, a number of criteria can be derived for critical evaluations of experimental mixture studies. First, the effects of individual mixture components ideally will be determined in parallel with the mixture experiment for the same end point. In some published studies, that was not done, and single-agent data from similar experimental conditions had to be relied on. Second, in well-designed studies, PODs are estimated for each mixture component, and the absence of statistically significant effects is verified by direct testing. Where that demand was not met, doses without significant effects had to be estimated by regression analysis of dose-response data on the individual chemicals based on similar conditions.

Mixture Effects of Combinations of Phthalates and Other Antiandrogens at Doses around Points of Departure

The study by Hass et al. (2007) was designed to assess low-dose-mixture effects of AR antagonists in a developmental-toxicity model in the rat. NOAELs for vinclozolin, flutamide, and procymidone were estimated with change in AGD as the end point. The NOAELs in the study were similar to BMDs corresponding to effect levels of about 5%. When all three chemicals were combined at doses equivalent to their own NOAELs, reductions in AGD of 50% were observed. Quantitatively, the effects agreed well with the responses predicted by dose addition (see Figure 5-3), and the results were supported by a statistical evaluation of the observed data with dose-additivity predictions.

Although not designed for such purposes, the experiment by Howdeshell et al. (2008) on suppression of testosterone synthesis after developmental exposure to five phthalates indicates that phthalates are able to work together when present at individually ineffective doses. Statistically significant reductions in fetal testosterone synthesis were observed after administration of a total mixture to pregnant Sprague-Dawley rats at 260 mg/kg-d. The mixture contained DPP at 20 mg/kg-d and each other phthalate at 60 mg/kg-d. DPP was tested on its own at 25 mg/kg-d, and the remaining phthalates were examined after single administration at 100 mg/kg-d. At those doses, none of the single phthalates induced effects significantly different from those recorded in unexposed controls,[2] although the doses in the single-phthalate experiments exceeded those in the mixture. Figure 5-4 extends the analysis to phthalate doses that were present in the lowest tested mixture dose of 260 mg/kg-d. That mixture dose produced a reduction in testosterone synthesis that was statistically significantly different from untreated controls. Regression analysis of the dose-response data on the individual phthalates was used by the committee to estimate BMDs and BMDLs (see Appendix C). The BMDL for BBP was estimated as 66 mg/kg-d. Those values were 20 mg/kg-d for DBP, 31 mg/kg-d for DEHP, 10 mg/kg-d for DPP, and 47

---

[2]A simultaneous test of equivalence between the unexposed controls and low doses (100 mg/kg-d for BBP, DBP, DEHP, and DINP and 25 mg/kg-d for DPP) was rejected; this indicated equivalence between the low-dose mean and the control mean according to a 35% rule for equivalence bounds for the ratio of means. The doses in the mixture of 260 mg/kg-d included BBP, DBP, DEHP, and DIBP at 60 mg/kg-d and DPP at 20 mg/kg-d (that is, at doses below those used in the equivalence test).

mg/kg-d for DIBP. Those BMDLs approach the doses present in the mixture of 260 mg/kg-d, which yielded statistically significant effects. The committee notes that dose-addition and independent-action predictions were generally similar, although dose addition gave the more conservative predictions (see also Figure 5-1).

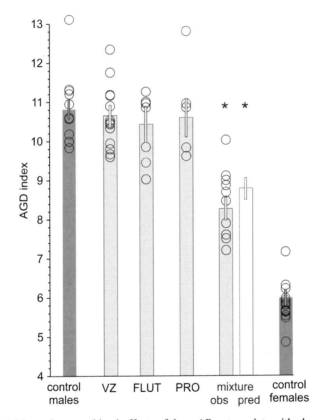

FIGURE 5-3 Low-dose combined effects of three AR antagonists with changes in AGD as the end point (Hass et al. 2007). Shown are litter means (circles) and mean responses with their 95% confidence intervals (bars with error bars). In all groups, the number of dams was 16, except for FLUT and PRO, in which case eight dams were dosed. When given as individual chemicals, vinclozolin (VZ, 24.5 mg/kg), flutamide (FLUT, 0.77 mg/kg), and prochloraz (PRO, 14.1 mg/kg) did not produce changes significantly differ-ent from those in control males. When combined at those doses (light gray bar, mixture obs), significant effects were observed (p < 0.05) that agreed well with the dose-addition prediction (white bar, mixture pred). NOAELs were estimated by using multiple contrast tests according to Hothorn (2004). The predicted mixture effects were derived from dose-response regression models for individual chemicals by using dose addition.

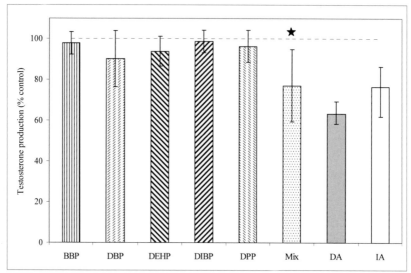

FIGURE 5-4 Low-dose combined effects of phthalates with suppression of testosterone synthesis as the end point. Shown is the committee's analysis of the data reported by Howdeshell et al. (2008). The hatched bars depict the model-predicted mean effects of BBP, DBP, DEHP, and DIBP at 60 mg/kg-d and DPP at 20 mg/kg-d. Error bars show 95% confidence intervals. Given the experimental design of Howdeshell et al., no individual mean effects would be predicted to be statistically distinguishable from controls (100% dotted line). The mean effect of a mixture of all phthalates at those doses (dotted bar, Mix) is statistically significantly different from untreated controls (the error bar shows the 99% confidence interval of the observed difference between mix and control groups). The expected mean combined effects derived from dose addition (DA, white bar) and independent action (IA, dark gray bar) are also shown, with 95% confidence intervals of the predicted mean. The individual responses to BBP, DBP, DEHP, and DIBP at 60 mg/kg-d and DPP at 20 mg/kg-d were estimated by fitting a nonlinear logistic regression model to the data reported by Howdeshell et al. (see Appendix C). Individual group means were obtained by applying the statistical model in Appendix C independently to each dose or control group. All confidence intervals were obtained with the profile likelihood method.

The study by Rider et al. (2008) provides some indications of combined effects of phthalates and AR antagonists at low doses. A combination of vinclozolin and procymidone (each at 3.75 mg/kg), prochloraz (8.75 mg/kg), linuron (5 mg/kg), and BBP, DBP, and DEHP (each at 37.5 mg/kg) was the lowest tested mixture dose that produced observable changes in AGD. Although the dose-response data on the individual chemicals are of insufficient quality to derive doses without observable effects, they nevertheless suggest that the doses are ineffective on their own. Similar conclusions can be drawn from the data provided for effects on NR and on hypospadias.

NON-DOSE-ADDITIVE COMBINED EFFECTS OF PHTHALATES AND OTHER ANTIANDROGENS

Strong evidence of non-dose-additive combined effects suggestive of synergism (relative to dose addition) with phthalates and other antiandrogens is lacking. However, there are some data that indicate toxic interactions (greater than dose-additive effects) when hypospadias and other genital malformations are evaluated as the end points of concern. Rider et al. (2008) found that BBP, DBP, DEHP, vinclozolin, procymidone, linuron, and prochloraz induced more hypospadias than predicted on the basis of dose addition. Because of the assumptions that had to be made in their study to bridge some data gaps (see above), it is not possible to say with certainty whether the observations represent a true synergism with respect to dose addition, but the possibility cannot be ruled out. To resolve the issue, it will be important to subject the individual chemicals and their combinations to extensive dose-response studies that specifically investigate hypospadias and other genital malformations.

Hotchkiss et al. (2004) tested a combination of BBP and linuron at doses that were ineffective on their own. When they were combined at the given doses, hypospadias, cleft phallus, and other genital malformations were found in about 60% of the male offspring. An assessment of the results in terms of deviation from expected additivity is complicated by the lack of dose-response data on the individual chemicals. Such an analysis would reveal whether the observed massive increases in malformations represent synergism or are the consequence of the low-dose additive effects previously discussed. The frequent extreme steepness of dose-response curves for hypospadias makes the latter explanation plausible.

Similar considerations apply to the results presented by Christiansen et al. (2008). About 50% of the male offspring showed genital malformations after exposure to a mixture of vinclozolin, flutamide, and procymidone, whereas none individually produced observable genital malformations at the doses used in the mixture as measured under the same conditions for vinclozolin and procymidone and on the basis of published data on flutamide.

The potential for non-dose-additive combined effects to occur should be systematically explored. The work should not only focus on combinations of phthalates and other antiandrogens but consider the possibility that chemicals devoid of antiandrogenic activity—for example, chemicals associated with testicular toxicity, such as cadmium—may exacerbate mixture effects.

CUMULATIVE RISK ASSESSMENT OF PHTHALATES AND OTHER ANTIANDROGENS: BASIC ISSUES

Cumulative risk assessment of phthalates and other antiandrogens cannot be implemented without addressing a number of basic issues. The first is the question of which chemicals to include in mixture risk assessment. The second is the mixture-effect assessment methods that can accurately predict combined effects. The third is the effects on which cumulative risk assessment should be based.

Which Criteria Should Be Used to Group Phthalates and Other Chemicals for Cumulative Risk Assessment?

The criterion proposed by EPA (2000) for grouping chemicals for cumulative risk assessment is "toxicological similarity," which may introduce ambiguities when applied to phthalates and other antiandrogens. An inappropriately narrow interpretation would exclude many chemicals that also produce effects related to the androgen-insufficiency syndrome.

Instead, a physiologically based approach for establishing grouping criteria for phthalates and other antiandrogens is strongly recommended. The recognition that androgen action is the driver of male sexual differentiation during development, with a multitude of underlying molecular mechanisms, implies that phenomenologic criteria should be used for grouping purposes. Thus, the starting point of approaches for grouping should be the physiologic process, not mechanisms or modes of action of the chemicals to be assessed. On the basis of considerations of the physiologic processes, a number of relevant end effects suggest themselves, and these should provide the basis of grouping. Accordingly, all chemicals that can induce some or all of the effects that make up the androgen-insufficiency syndrome should be subjected to cumulative risk assessment. Table 5-2 lists examples of chemicals that should be grouped with phthalates and considered for cumulative risk assessment.

TABLE 5-2 Examples of Chemicals That Should Be Considered for Cumulative Risk Assessment of Phthalates and Other Antiandrogens According to a Physiologically Based Grouping Approach

Chemical	End Point or Evidence
Phthalates: BBP, DBP, DEHP, DIBP, DINP, DPP	Androgen-insufficiency syndrome, testosterone-dependent development
AR antagonists: vinclozolin, procymidone	Androgen-insufficiency syndrome, dihydrotestosterone-dependent development
Linuron, prochloraz	Androgen-insufficiency syndrome, AR antagonists, suppression of testosterone synthesis
5α-reductase inhibitors	Androgen-insufficiency syndrome, dihydrotestosterone-dependent development
Azole fungicides: ketoconazole, tebuconazole, propiconazole	Suppression of testosterone synthesis in vivo, AGD changes in vivo
Polybrominated diphenyl ethers	AR antagonists in vivo
TCDD, some PCBs	Suppression of AR expression, AGD changes in vivo

There are reports that 2,3,7,8-tetrachloro-dibenzo-*p*-dioxin (TCDD) can induce reductions in AGD by a mechanism that involves down-regulation of the AR and consequent suppression of AR-dependent genes in reproductive tissues (Ohsako et al. 2002). Reductions in AGD have also been observed with some coplanar polychlorinated biphenyls (PCBs) (Faqi et al. 1998; Rice 1999). Thus, a physiologic approach to grouping antiandrogens for purposes of cumulative risk assessment suggests inclusion of those chemicals. In contrast, the remaining effects typically attributed to the androgen-insufficiency syndrome, such as changes in NR and malformations, have not been found after administration of dioxins or PCBs in reproductive developmental-toxicity studies of rodents. Experimental studies are needed to resolve the issue of combined effects of TCDD, PCBs, and other antiandrogens.

Which Approach Should Be Used for Quantifying Cumulative Risks Posed by Phthalates and Other Chemicals?

The brief overview of relevant mixture studies of antiandrogens has shown that there is strong empirical evidence of dose addition as an accurate predictor of mixture effects. Independent action often yielded similar quantitative predictions but in some cases has led to substantial underestimation of combined effects. The committee could identify no case in which independent action predicted combined effects that were in agreement with experimentally observed responses and at the same time were larger than the effects anticipated by using dose addition.

Because the use of relative potencies and the use of TEFs are special applications of the dose-addition concept, such approaches might suggest themselves as a straightforward way of making quantitative assessments of the effects of phthalates and other antiandrogens. However, application of the relative-potency concept (and a fortiori the TEF concept) requires parallel dose-response curves. If that demand is not met, equivalence factors will vary with the effect levels chosen for analysis. The data provided by Hass et al. (2007), Metzdorff et al. (2007), Howdeshell et al. (2008), and Rider et al. (2008) show clearly that phthalates and antiandrogens exhibit dose-response curves with widely differing slopes and shapes. An additional complication is the fact that dose-response relationships vary widely with the end point chosen for analysis. The relative potency of antiandrogens is not the same for every end point, so it is difficult to assign a global TEF to a specific antiandrogen. Thus, basic requirements for using either the relative-potency or TEF approach are violated, and their use cannot be recommended.

Instead, dose addition should be used for quantitative evaluations of the joint effects of phthalates and other antiandrogens. It is a widely held misconception (EPA 2000) that dose addition is applicable only with congruent dose-response curves (for a general discussion, see Gennings et al. 2005 and Kortenkamp et al. 2007). Although high-quality dose-response data on individual chemicals are desirable as a basis of predictions about mixture effects over a range of effect levels, dose addition can also be used when only point estimates, such as NOAELs, are available.

Defining Points of Departure for Mixtures

A mixture that produces dose-additive effects must satisfy the following expression:

$$\sum_{i=1}^{n} \frac{c_i{}^*}{ECx_i} = 1, \tag{1}$$

where $c_i{}^*$ is the concentration (or dose) of substance i in a mixture that produces a known total effect X and ECx_i is the concentration (or dose) of substance i that causes the effect X when applied individually. When the sum of the terms is larger than 1, there is antagonism; when it is smaller than 1, there is synergism. Equation 1 is referred to as the sum of toxic units or the sum of hazard indexes for particular selections of ECx_i, such as reference doses.

The schematic in Figure 5-5 illustrates how the interrelations play out when the aim is to establish a POD for a mixture of five hypothetical chemicals. In this example, the thin vertical lines associated with the individual dose-response curves in Figure 5-5 represent the BMDLs for each single chemical. Let the BMDLs corresponding to a particular benchmark response (BMR) of chemicals 1-5 be 90, 3.5, 11.8, 17.8, and 3.95 mg/kg-d, respectively. By using dose addition, it is possible to predict the effects of a mixture of all five chemicals when the mixture ratios are in proportion to the individual BMDLs (black solid curve in Figure 5-5). The black curve can be used to read off the expected effect of a dose of the mixture equal to the sum of all BMDLs. That procedure shows that the combination of the BMDLs cannot be considered to be without effect because it produces a reduction in response to about 90% in this particular case (black dashed vertical and horizontal arrows in Figure 5-5). To ensure that the mixture effect of the five chemicals is indistinguishable from the effect associated with the BMDLs of the individual chemicals, the doses of the mixture components have to be lowered.

Equation 1 can be used to determine how much lower the doses of all individual components of the mixture must be to ensure that the combined effect corresponds to the BMR. That will occur when Equation 1 is fulfilled for the special case of $ECx_i = BMDL_i$. Several permutations of the doses $c_i{}^*$ of the chemicals in the mixture that satisfy Equation 1 can be found. One can distinguish the following two extremes:

(1) A single chemical is present at its BMDL. Equation 1 holds only when the doses of all other chemicals are zero.

(2) Equation 1 holds when all chemicals are present at their individual BMDLs divided by the number of the other effective chemicals in the combination, five in the present example. Thus, with the individual BMDLs of chemicals 1-5 of 90, 3.5, 11.8, 17.8 and 3.95 mg/kg-d, respectively, Equation 1 holds with $(90/5)/90 + (3.5/5)/3.5 + (11.8/5)/11.8 + (17.8/5)/17.8 + (3.95/5)/3.95$, which resolves to $1/5 + 1/5 + 1/5 + 1/5 + 1/5 = 1$. In other words, a combination of chemicals 1-5 of 18, 0.7, 2.36, 3.56, and 0.79 mg/kg-d, respectively, should produce less than the BMR (black vertical arrow in Figure 5-5).

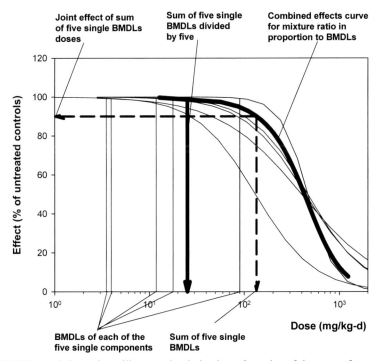

FIGURE 5-5 Schematic to illustrate the derivation of a point of departure for a mixture dose, here the lower confidence limit of a benchmark dose (BMDL). Shown are the dose-response curves for five single hypothetical chemicals (thin curves) and their corresponding BMDLs (thin vertical lines). In this hypothetical case, 100% equals the effect seen in untreated controls. The solid black curve shows the combined effects of a mixture of all five chemicals with mixture ratios proportional to their individual BMDLs. The sum of the single BMDLs (vertical dashed arrow) will exceed the effect associated with the BMDLs, the so-called benchmark response (horizontal black dashed arrow). To achieve the benchmark response for the mixture (black vertical arrow), the individual BMDLs of all components have to be lowered by a factor of 5. Other combinations may also reach a combined zero effect, and these are accessible by calculating new mixture effect curves corresponding to the chosen mixture ratios. If one component is present at its BMDL, the mixture is without effect only when the doses of all other components are zero.

The example presented here can be extended to the case where all chemicals are present in an arbitrary mixture. In that case, the sum in Equation 1 will be less than 1 provided that every chemical is present at less than its BMDL/n, so that in all cases such a mixture will have an effect less than the BMR.

When the aim is to assess the effects of joint existing exposures, the procedure is slightly different. Equation 1 can be used, but this time with c_i^* representing the doses of the individual chemicals that are in specific exposure scenarios. As before, ECx_i represents the individual BMDLs of each chemical i. If the sum of the toxic units c_i^*/ECx_i is less than 1, the joint effect of the mixture must be less than the BMR at least under the dose-addition hypothesis.

Which Effect Outcomes Should Form the Basis of Cumulative Risk Assessment?

PODs, such as BMDs and NOAELs, for individual chemicals in mixtures are important elements of cumulative risk assessment. They can be the basis of reference values for cumulative effects, which can be used for risk assessment or standard-setting. Reference values for individual chemicals are estimated in relation to specific effect outcomes and toxic end points. However, although the specific effects produced by phthalates and other antiandrogens show commonalities, there are differences. The responses seen after disruption of androgen action during development depend on whether the effects of dihydrotestosterone or those of testosterone are compromised. Although there is overlap in the spectrum of effects resulting from exposure to phthalates and other antiandrogens, some responses are specific to disruption of testosterone action, and others are seen only after blocking of dihydrotestosterone action. For example, none of the AR antagonists suppresses testosterone synthesis, and they have weaker effects in disrupting the development of testosterone-dependent tissues, such as the epididymis. Conversely, phthalates are less effective in disrupting reproductive development that depends on dihydrotestosterone and causing malformations, such as hypospadias, that result from that type of disruption.

To make a common grouping of phthalates and other antiandrogens practicable, it is necessary to deal with the fact that not all relevant agents produce all aspects of the androgen-insufficiency syndrome. The committee has considered several ways of addressing that situation. One option is to recognize that the induction of any of the effects of the androgen-insufficiency syndrome is symptomatic of disruption of androgen action. Therefore, the androgen-insufficiency syndrome should be dealt with as a whole. This approach makes it necessary to aggregate the various qualitatively different components of the syndrome into one common measure. Because the array of effects produced by phthalates and other antiandrogens shows a degree of overlap, an alternative option is to focus on effects common to the chemicals and to base cumulative risk assessment on the most sensitive common outcome. Those two options and their implications are detailed in the following sections.

Option 1: Dealing with the Syndrome as a Whole

The qualitatively different component effects of the androgen-insufficiency syndrome can be aggregated by noting for each experimental subject as to whether any of the observed end points signify some degree of toxicity. For example, one might say that any malformation, an AGD deviating by two standard deviations from the mean of that in the unexposed control group, or an organ weight below a specified weight would indicate that the subject experienced toxicity.[3] A usual analysis of dose-response data could then be conducted by using those measures of toxicity for each experimental subject. Although the method incorporates multiple end points associated with the androgen-insufficiency syndrome, it assumes equal levels of toxicity associated with each dichotomized end point in classifying each subject as demonstrating toxicity or not. In this way, PODs, such as BMDs and NOAELs, for single chemicals can be estimated and used as input for deriving reference values for combinations of antiandrogens.

A variation would be to develop a scoring method that incorporates the set of end points while adjusting for the degree of toxicity related to each end point. For example, a method commonly used in the engineering literature known as desirability functions (see Appendix D) could be used to define a toxicity score for each of the component end points of the syndrome on a unitless scale between 0 (most toxicity) and 1 (no toxicity). On the basis of each end-point-specific toxicity score, an overall composite toxicity score can be constructed. Coffey et al. (2007) have described the development of such an overall composite score for the many outcomes measured in toxicologic studies. Appendix D shows how this approach can be used productively for the assessment of antiandrogenic chemicals.

Option 2: Focusing on the Most Sensitive End Point of the Androgen-Insufficiency Syndrome

It appears that in neonatal male rats NR is the most sensitive common effect of phthalates, AR antagonists, and chemicals that act via a mixed mechanism of action. Thus, NR in rats could be chosen as a common end point, and the BMDs or NOAELs for single chemicals could form the basis of cumulative risk assessments of phthalates and other antiandrogens.

However, phthalates induce reductions in testosterone synthesis at lower doses than required for changes in NR. Therefore, risks posed by phthalates might be underestimated if cumulative risk assessment is conducted in relation to NR in rats. Comparative dose-response studies would need to be conducted to

---

[3]The committee is not endorsing any specific value to signify toxicity; that is a matter for further evaluation.

evaluate the degree to which hazard assessments based on NR in rats could underestimate the risks associated with phthalates.

If the use of NR in rats as the evaluation end point is insufficiently protective, the most sensitive individual end point for each of the groups of antiandrogens (for example, reduction in testosterone synthesis for phthalates or NR for AR antagonists) could be chosen for the estimation of reference values, which in turn are used to derive cumulative effects as a sum of toxic units or hazard indexes. However, this approach violates one of the preconditions of dose addition—the induction of the same effect. Nevertheless, it can be used from a pragmatic viewpoint, considering that there is a precedent for it in the use of hazard indexes.

Estimation of Cumulative Effects: Animal-to-Human Extrapolation

An issue for consideration with the above options is whether aggregation for cumulative effects should be conducted with animal data and then extrapolated to the human or whether reference values for human exposure, such as a tolerable daily intake (TDI), should be derived first for individual chemicals and aggregation for cumulative risks then carried out with TDIs in a second step. Those alternatives are depicted schematically in Figure 5-6.

The first approach (Figure 5-6A) is suitable for almost all the options outlined above for dealing with the different end points of the androgen-insufficiency syndrome except perhaps when the most sensitive individual end point is used to derive reference values for single chemicals. In that case, it might be more appropriate to estimate TDIs first (Figure 5-6A); this allows additional flexibility by giving the opportunity to adopt tailor-made uncertainty factors for each individual chemical during the estimation of single chemical TDIs. Because the aggregation for cumulative effects is carried out with individual TDIs, the use of different end points from animal studies for the estimation of TDIs can be accommodated. The procedure sketched in Figure 5-6B is also compatible with all the options for dealing with the component effects of the androgen-insufficiency syndrome that were discussed above.

STEPPED APPROACHES TO CUMULATIVE RISK ASSESSMENT OF PHTHALATES AND OTHER ANTIANDROGENS

A corollary of the dose-addition principle is that cumulative effects are to be expected even when all mixture components are present at doses below their zero effect levels for the individual components if a sufficiently high number of relevant chemicals are combined at sufficient doses. The demonstration that exposure to individual chemicals may be below some risk-criterion level for the individual components is uninformative. To estimate risks that stem from cumulative exposure to phthalates and other antiandrogens, information on the nature

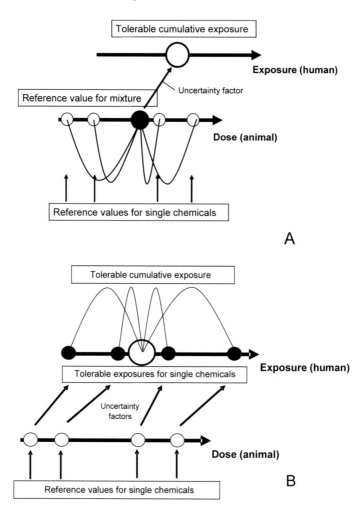

FIGURE 5-6 Aggregation for cumulative effects and animal-to-human extrapolation. The horizontal black arrows represent dose axes for the effects of antiandrogens in animals and humans. (A) Aggregation for cumulative effects (large black circle on "dose [animal]" axis) is carried out at the level of animal-derived reference values (open small circles on "dose [animal]" axis). The calculation of mixture effects is symbolized by the parabolic lines. A reference value for cumulative effects in animals (black circle) is then combined with an uncertainty factor to derive tolerable cumulative exposures for humans (large white circle on "exposure [human]" axis). (B) Reference values for single chemicals (open small circles on "dose [animal]" axis) are combined with uncertainty factors to derive individual tolerable exposures for humans first (black circles on "dose [human]" axis); these values are then used to derive standards for cumulative risk assessment (large white circle on "dose [human]" axis).

of the chemicals in the mixture, the magnitude of exposures to the individual chemicals, their potency, and their number is required. Thus, knowledge about the prevalence and quantities of other chemicals that might contribute to the risk in question is critical. Incomplete information about this aspect of exposure assessment will introduce considerable uncertainty and the potential for underestimating risks.

The example illustrated in Figure 5-5 highlights the ways in which the presence of other chemicals that produce the effect of interest determines the extent to which threshold levels for single compounds may have to be corrected to ensure that a mixture is without effect. The larger the number of effective chemicals, the larger the downward correction of the single thresholds may have to be to guarantee safety. What is the number of antiandrogens that might contribute to disrupting male sexual differentiation?

Recent screening efforts for AR antagonists provide some first clues. Kojima et al. (2004) examined 200 pesticides for their ability to antagonize the AR. Of the 200 tested compounds, 66 were found to be active. Vinggaard et al. (2008) screened 397 chemicals for AR antagonism and identified 178 active ones, of which 17 had a potency higher than or similar to that of flutamide. The authors developed a global quantitative structure-activity-relationship model that predicted that 8% of the chemicals would be active AR antagonists.

Those efforts suggest that a large number of chemicals might be active in vivo AR antagonists capable of disrupting male sexual differentiation. Possibly because of toxicokinetic influences that prevent the buildup of suitably high concentrations in target tissues, some in vitro antagonists fail to show effects in in vivo models. However, insufficient information is available about correlations between in vitro and in vivo antiandrogens. Conclusive data that might help to resolve the issue are not likely to become available soon, not least because the testing of candidate chemicals in in vivo developmental-toxicity models is extremely time-consuming and expensive.

The uncertainties and knowledge gaps call for appropriately conservative approaches that incorporate default assumptions about the likely number of antiandrogens that might contribute to human exposure scenarios. The committee's proposal to deal with that would be adoption of a stepped approach as follows.

Step 1: Cumulative Risk Assessment with Incorporation of Default Assumptions about the Likely Number and Potency of Unidentified Antiandrogens

In a first screening step, cumulative risk assessment of phthalates, AR antagonists, and mixed-mode antiandrogens could be carried out by making allowance for unidentified antiandrogens. That could be achieved by using the toxic unit (hazard index) Equation 1, as follows: Human exposures to each chemical are represented by c_i^*, and ECx_i are estimates of tolerable daily exposures. To take account of unidentified antiandrogens of unknown potency, a default number of "placeholder" toxic units (for example, 10-100) can be added. That requires some assumptions about the potency and prevalence of the unknowns. A reasonable first approximation would be to expect ECx_i around the median of the TDIs for established in vivo antiandrogens, with c_i* equal to ECx_i divided by the total number of toxic units in the equation.

If the sum of toxic units obtained in this way is 1 or smaller, the cumulative risks posed by phthalates and related chemicals can be regarded as quite low.

If, however, the procedure yields a value larger than 1, risk-reduction measures may be advised. Alternatively, the assessment can be refined.

Step 2: Cumulative Risk Assessment of Phthalates and Other Antiandrogens

The above procedure is repeated by including AR antagonists and mixed-mode antiandrogens that have known in vivo activity but without making assumptions about unidentified antiandrogens. If this step signals risks, risk-reduction measures may have to be considered. Alternatively, a refined step considering only phthalates may be included.

It is also possible to conduct the stepwise procedure in reverse order, beginning with phthalates and antiandrogens that have established in vivo activity. If the first risk-assessment step does not indicate risks, the assessment broadens to assume worse-case scenarios.

STANDARD-SETTING

In some regulatory settings, it may be deemed desirable to derive exposure standards for phthalates and other antiandrogens that take account of cumulative exposures. In such cases, tolerable daily exposures to individual chemicals could be corrected downward by incorporating an additional "mixture uncertainty factor." The additional uncertainty factor would have to take account of the number of chemicals to which simultaneous effective coexposure is deemed likely.

CONCLUSIONS

A major challenge to conducting cumulative risk assessment is choosing an approach to predict mixture effects. However, evidence from the recent peer-reviewed scientific literature shows not only that phthalates produce mixture effects but that the effects are often predicted well by using the dose-addition concept. That is also true for other classes of antiandrogens and for combinations of phthalates with such antiandrogens. Although a variety of molecular mechanisms are at play, dose addition provided equal or better approximations of mixture effects compared with independent action (when such comparisons were performed). In no example in the literature did independent action produce a mixture-effect prediction that proved to be correct and differed substantially from that produced with dose addition. The evidence that supports adoption of a physiologic approach is strong. Experimental evidence demonstrates that toxic effects of phthalates and other antiandrogens are similar despite differences in the molecular details of the mechanisms, including metabolism, distribution, and elimination.

The criteria recommended by EPA (2000) for guiding decisions between dose addition and independent action appear too narrow when applied to phthalates and other antiandrogens, particularly those requiring similarity in uptake, metabolism, distribution, and elimination and congruent dose-response curves for application of dose addition. The requirements are not met by combinations of phthalates with other antiandrogens, but the dose-addition principle applies. The case for using dose addition as an approximation for mixture risk assessment of phthalates and other antiandrogens is strong.

When risks posed by low-level exposures need to be evaluated, there are substantial differences between the single-chemical approach and cumulative risk assessment. There is good evidence that combinations of phthalates and of other antiandrogens produce combined effects at doses that when administered alone do not have significant effects. In some cases, those doses are similar to those used as PODs to estimate tolerable human exposure. The results highlight the problem that may arise when PODs for individual chemicals are used as the basis of human-health risk assessment in situations in which exposure to other chemicals with similar effects also occurs. The results emphasize the necessity of conducting cumulative risk assessment of phthalates and other antiandrogens to assess risks posed by exposure to mixtures of these compounds. Assessments based solely on the effects of single phthalates and other antiandrogens may lead to considerable underestimation of risks to the developing fetus.

In this chapter, the committee has provided recommendations on various aspects of conducting cumulative risk assessment. The recommendations were designed specifically to deal with phthalates and antiandrogens. However, the conceptual framework that the committee has used is generic and lends itself to dealing with other groups of chemicals, provided that the relevant toxicologic data are available.

REFERENCES

Allen, B.C., R.J. Kavlock, C.A. Kimmel, and E.M. Faustman. 1994. Dose-response assessment for developmental toxicity. II. Comparison of generic benchmark dose estimates with no observed adverse effect levels. Fundam. Appl. Toxicol. 23(4):487-495.

Berenbaum, M.C. 1989. What is synergy? Pharmacol Rev. 41(2):93-141.

Bility, M.T., J.T. Thompson, R.H. McKee, R.M. David, J.H. Butala, J.P. Vanden Heuvel, and J.M. Peters. 2004. Activation of mouse and human peroxisome proliferator-activated receptors (PPARs) by phthalate monoesters. Toxicol. Sci. 82(1):170-182.

Birkhoj, M., C. Nellemann, K. Jarfelt, H. Jacobsen, H.R. Andersen, M. Dalgaard, and A.M. Vinggaard. 2004. The combined antiandrogenic effects of five commonly used pesticides. Toxicol. Appl. Pharmacol. 201(1):10-20.

Christiansen, S., M. Scholze, M. Axelstad, J. Boberg, A. Kortenkamp, and U. Hass. 2008. Combined exposure to anti-androgens causes markedly increased frequencies of hypospadias in the rat. Int. J. Androl. 31(2):241-248.

Coffey, J., C. Gennings, and V.M. Moser. 2007. The simultaneous analysis of discrete and continuous outcomes in a dose-response study: Using desirability functions. Regul. Toxicol. Pharmacol. 48(1):51-58.

COT (Committee on Toxicity of Chemicals in Food, Consumer Products and the Environment). 2002. Risk Assessment of Mixtures of Pesticides and Similar Substances. London, UK: Her Majesty's Stationary Office [online]. Available: http://cot.food.gov.uk/pdfs/reportindexed.pdf [accessed 28 June 2008].

Crump, K.S. 1984. A new method for determining allowable daily intakes. Fundam. Appl. Toxicol. 4(5):854-871.

Crump, K.S. 2002. Critical issues in benchmark calculations from continuous data. Crit. Rev. Toxicol. 32(3):133-153.

EPA (U.S. Environmental Protection Agency). 1986. Guidelines for the Health Risk Assessment of Chemical Mixtures. EPA/630/R-98/002. Risk Assessment Forum, U.S. Environmental Protection Agency, Washington, DC. September 1986 [online]. Available: http://www.epa.gov/ncea/raf/pdfs/chem_mix/chemmix_1986.pdf [accessed July 23, 2008].

EPA (U.S. Environmental Protection Agency). 1989. Risk Assessment Guidance for Superfund, Volume I. Human Health Evaluation Manual (Part A). Interim Final. EPA/540/1-89/002. PB90-155581. Office of Emergency and Remedial Response, U.S. Environmental Protection Agency, Washington, DC. December 1989 [online]. Available: http://rais.ornl.gov/homepage/HHEMA.pdf [accessed July 22, 2008].

EPA (U.S. Environmental Protection Agency). 1994. Methods for Derivation of Inhalation Reference Concentrations and Application of Inhalation Dosimetry. EPA/600/8-90/066F. Office of Research and Development, U.S. Environmental Protection Agency, Washington, DC [online]. Available: http://cfpub.epa.gov/ncea/cfm/recordisplay.cfm?deid=71993 [accessed Oct. 16, 2008].

EPA (U.S. Environmental Protection Agency). 2000. Supplementary Guidance for Conducting Health Risk Assessment of Chemical Mixtures. EPA/630/R-00/002. Risk Assessment Forum, U.S. Environmental Protection Agency, Washington, DC. August 2000 [online]. Available: http://www.epa.gov/NCEA/raf/pdfs/chem_mix/chem_mix_08_2001.pdf [accessed June 10, 2008].

EPA (U.S. Environmental Protection Agency). 2002. Guidance on Cumulative Risk Assessment of Pesticide Chemicals That Have a Common Mechanism of Toxicity. Office of Pesticide Programs, U.S. Environmental Protection Agency, Washington, DC. January 14, 2002 [online]. Available: http://www.epa.gov/oppfead1/trac/science/cumulative_guidance.pdf [accessed June 10, 2008].

Faqi, A.S., P.R. Dalsenter, H.J. Merker, and I. Chahoud. 1998. Effects on developmental landmarks and reproductive capability of 3, 3', 4,4'-tetrachlorobiphenyl and 3,3'4,4',5-pentachlorobiphenyl in offspring of rats exposed during pregnancy. Hum. Exp. Toxicol. 17(7):365-372.

Foster, P.M. 2005. Mode of action: Impaired fetal Leydig cell function – effects on male reproductive development produced by certain phthalate esters. Crit. Rev. Toxicol. 35(8-9):713-719.

Gennings, C., W.H. Carter Jr., R.A. Carchman, L.K. Teuschler, J.E. Simmons, and E.W. Carney. 2005. A unifying concept for assessing toxicological interactions: Changes in slope. Toxicol. Sci. 88(2):287-297.

Gray, L.E., J. Ostby, J. Furr, C. J. Wolf, C. Lambright, L. Parks, D.N. Veeramachaneni, V. Wilson, M. Price, A. Hotchkiss, E. Orlando, and L. Guilette. 2001. Effects of environmental antiandorgens on reproductive development in experimental animals. Hum. Reprod. Update 7(3):248-264.

Hass, U., M. Scholze, S. Christiansen, M. Dalgaard, A.M. Vinggaard, M. Axelstad, S.B. Metzdorff, and A. Kortenkamp. 2007. Combined exposure to anti-androgens exacerbates disruption of sexual differentiation in the rat. Environ. Health Perspect. 115 (Suppl. 1):122-128.

Hotchkiss, A.K, L.G. Parks-Saldutti, J.S. Ostby, C. Lambright, J. Furr, J.G. Vandenbergh, and L.E. Gray Jr. 2004. A mixture of the "antiandrogens" linuron and butyl benzyl phthalate alters sexual differentiation of the male rat in a cumulative fashion. Biol. Reprod. 71(6):1852-1861.

Hothorn, L. 2004. A robust statistical procedure for evaluating genotoxicity data. Environmetrics 15(6):635-641.

Howdeshell, K.L., J. Furr, C.R. Lambright, C.V. Rider, V.S. Wilson, and L.E. Gray Jr. 2007. Cumulative effects of dibutyl phthalate and diethylhexyl phthalate on male rat reproductive tract development: Altered fetal steroid hormones and genes. Toxicol. Sci. 99(1):190-202.

Howdeshell, K.L., V.S. Wilson, J. Furr, C.R. Lambright, C.V. Rider, C.R. Blystone, A.K. Hotchkiss, and L.E. Gray, Jr. 2008. A mixture of five phthalate esters inhibits fetal testicular testosterone production in the Sprague-Dawley rat in a cumulative, dose-additive manner. Toxicol. Sci. 105(1):153-165.

Kojima, H., E. Katsura, S. Takeuchi, K. Niyama, and K. Kobayashi. 2004. Screening for estrogen and androgen receptor activities in 200 pesticides by in vitro reporter gene assays using Chinese hamster ovary cells. Environ. Health Perspect. 112(5):524-531.

Kortenkamp, A., M. Faust, M. Scholze, and T. Backhaus. 2007. Low level exposure to multiple chemicals: Reason for human health concerns? Environ. Health Perspect. 115(Suppl. 1):106-114.

Loewe, S., and H. Muischnek. 1926. Über Kombinationswirkungen I. Mitteilung: Hilfsmittel der Fragestellung. N-S. Arch. Exp. Pathol. Pharmakol. 114:313-326.

Metzdorff, S.B., M. Dalgaard, S. Christiansen, M. Axelstad, U. Hass, M.K. Kiersgaard, M. Scholze, A. Kortenkamp, and A.M. Vinggaard. 2007. Dysgenesis and histological changes of genitals and perturbations of gene expression in male rats after in utero exposure to antiandrogen mixtures. Toxicol. Sci. 98(1):87-98.

Mileson, B.E., J.E. Chambers, W.L. Chen, W. Dettbarn, M. Ehrich, A.T. Eldefrawi, D.W. Gaylor, K. Hamernik, E. Hodgson, A.G. Karczmar, S. Padilla, C.N. Pope, R.J. Richardson, D.R. Saunders, L.P. Sheets, L.G. Sultatos, and K.B. Wallace. 1998. Common mechanism of toxicity: A case study of organophosphorus pesticides. Toxicol. Sci. 41(1):8-20.

Nellemann, C., M. Dalgaard, H.R. Lam, and A.M. Vinggaard. 2003. The combined effects of vinclozolin and procymidone do not deviate from expected additivity in vitro and in vivo. Toxicol. Sci. 71(2):251-262.

NRC (National Research Council). 2000. Toxicological Effects of Methylmercury. Washington, DC: National Academy Press.

Ohsako, S., Y. Miyabara, M. Sakane, R. Ishimura, M. Kakeyama, H. Izumi, J. Yonemoto, and C. Tohama. 2002. Developmental stage-specific effects of perinatal 2,3,7,8

TCDD exposure on reproductive organs of male rat offspring. Toxicol. Sci. 66(2):283-292.

Rice, C. 1999. Effect of exposure to 3, 3'4, 4',5-pentachlorobiphenyl (PCB 126) throughout gestation and lactation on development and spatial delayed alternation performance in rats. Neurotoxicol. Teratol. 21(1):59-69.

Rider, C.V., J. Furr, V.S. Wilson, and L.E. Gray Jr. 2008. A mixture of seven antiandrogens induces reproductive malformations in rats. Int. J. Androl. 31(2):249-262.

Scholze, M., and A. Kortenkamp. 2007. Statistical power considerations show the endocrine disrupter low dose issue in a new light. Environ. Health Perspect. 115 (Suppl. 1):84-90.

Slob, W. 1999. Thresholds in toxicology and risk assessment. Int J. Toxicol. 18(4): 259-268.

Stroheker, T., N. Cabaton, G. Nourdin, J.F. Regnier, J.C. Lhuguenot, and M.C. Chagnon. 2005. Evaluation of anti-androgenic activity of di-(2-ethylhexyl)phthalate. Toxicology 208(1):115-121.

Vinggaard, A.M., J. Niemala, E.B. Wedebye, and G.E. Jensen. 2008. Screening of 397 chemicals and development of a quantitative structure-activity relationship model for androgen receptor antagonism. Chem. Res. Toxicol. 21(4):813-823.

6

Data Gaps and Research Needs

On review of the scientific literature on phthalates, the committee found that sufficient data are available to conduct a cumulative risk assessment of these chemicals. Accordingly, progress need not wait for data gaps identified here to be addressed. Instead, the research recommended will allow greater refinement of the cumulative risk assessment for all health outcomes associated with phthalates and reduce uncertainty associated with such an assessment.

EXPOSURE ASSESSMENT

As discussed in Chapter 2, phthalates are used in a wide variety of consumer products and building materials, and widespread exposure of the general population has been documented through the National Health and Nutrition Examination Surveys (NHANES) conducted by the Centers for Disease Control and Prevention. Research initiatives outlined below would answer important questions concerning human exposure and greatly refine any cumulative risk assessment of phthalates.

- Identify across the human life span the important sources of phthalate exposure and the migration pathways that connect the sources to members of the general population, including highly exposed or susceptible groups. Elucidate across the life span the proportional contributions of exposure media (such as toys, dust, air, food, and soil) and exposure routes (ingestion, inhalation, and dermal) and define which media and routes are most important. Define the degree to which phthalates are absorbed by the three exposure routes.
- Identify the full spectrum of phthalate metabolites, particularly the oxidized metabolites of DEHP and DINP; determine whether they differ by exposure route; and determine the most appropriate metabolites to use as biomarkers of human exposure and the most appropriate biologic matrices in which to measure them.
- Improve the understanding of metabolism and of how metabolism might change over a lifetime. For example, is metabolism in the fetus, infant, or child different from metabolism in adults?

- Determine the basis of differences observed in children's vs adults' urinary concentrations. For example, are the observed differences related to differences in exposure or to differences in metabolism?
- Determine prenatal exposure by using phthalate-exposure biomarkers (that is, urine and amniotic fluid) at multiple relevant times during pregnancy. It is especially important to determine whether the various metabolite concentrations vary with time; if so, it might indicate differences in metabolism according to gestational age.
- Determine the relationship between maternal urinary phthalate metabolite concentrations and those in the fetal compartment (for example, concentrations in amniotic fluid), with an emphasis on understanding the pharmacokinetics of phthalates in the fetal compartment.
- Characterize human exposure to other antiandrogens and other factors that contribute to disturbed androgen action. Determine the possibility of coexposure, in which case the chemicals would exhibit joint action.
- Use existing large databases, such as NHANES, to assess exposure to multiple phthalates and other chemicals that may contribute to common biologic outcomes. Incorporate state-of-the-art exposure-assessment strategies for multiple phthalates and other chemicals in large or planned epidemiologic studies, such as the National Children's Study.
- Develop pharmacokinetic models that can allow better predictions of human fetal exposure on the basis of animal studies.

TOXICITY ASSESSMENT

As discussed in Chapter 3, although few human data are available, rats exposed to a variety of phthalates have exhibited reproductive developmental effects that mirror the hypothesized testicular dysgenesis syndrome in humans. The research initiatives outlined below would add substantially to the scientific database and enable better prediction of effects of phthalate exposure.

- Conduct studies to determine whether there are multigenerational effects of specific phthalates, phthalate-antiandrogen mixtures, and antiandrogen mixtures that have not yet been tested.
- Elucidate the mechanisms of phthalate action in fetal vs adult tissue, mechanistic differences between species, and any potential for differences in effects related to exposure route.
- Determine whether in utero exposure combined with lifetime exposure affects the incidence and severity of cancer outcomes. As discussed in Chapter 3, hepatic, testicular, and pancreatic cancers have been associated with activation of the peroxisome-proliferator-activated receptor-α (PPARα), but there is evidence that these cancer types may be mediated by mechanisms independent of PPARα. Because fetuses and neonates may exhibit sensitivity to PPARα ligands different from that exhibited by adults and the majority of studies have

focused solely on adult animal models, it is important to determine whether in utero exposure affects cancer outcomes and, if so, by what mechanisms.

• Conduct epidemiologic studies to evaluate potential health outcomes of phthalate-antiandrogen exposures. Attempt to characterize and evaluate effects in susceptible or highly exposed groups. Confirm and extend current information on the relationship between anogenital distance and infant testosterone concentration.

• Conduct toxicity studies of phthalate metabolites to determine potential adverse effects associated with exposure to them.

CUMULATIVE RISK ASSESSMENT

As discussed in Chapter 5, available data support the appropriateness of cumulative risk assessment of phthalates and other antiandrogen compounds. Research initiatives that would refine such an assessment are outlined below.

• Explore combination effects of phthalates, other antiandrogens, and other endocrine-disrupting agents.
• Investigate deviations from additivity observed when hypospadias is used as the selected outcome.
• Refine estimates of composite scores for disruption of androgen action.
• Develop approaches to the epidemiologic assessment of the cumulative effects of phthalates and other antiandrogens.

DATA RESOURCES FOR CUMULATIVE RISK ASSESSMENT

The committee emphasizes that the quality of results of any risk assessment is based on the data available. The U.S. Environmental Protection Agency (EPA) Integrated Risk Information System (IRIS) is the source of much of the toxicity information used in risk assessment today. Many of the chemical profiles in IRIS need to be updated; the information is no longer relevant or accurate. The phthalate profiles available in IRIS illustrate that point. The committee recognizes that the task of profile review and revision is enormous; however, linking profiles to current literature would be helpful. For example, IRIS profiles of chemicals that also are the subject of interaction profiles produced by the Agency for Toxic Substances and Disease Registry would ideally be linked to the interaction profiles. Furthermore, as EPA moves toward cumulative risk assessment, some consideration should be given to restructuring IRIS so that its process for identifying chemicals for review includes and sets priorities among chemical mixtures, as appropriate, and facilitates cumulative risk assessment conducted by using common adverse outcomes. For example, listing the no-observed-adverse-effect levels or benchmark doses for a variety of effects would facilitate that approach.

Appendix A

Statement of Task

A National Research Council committee will evaluate human health risks and the potential for conducting a cumulative risk assessment for phthalate esters. The committee will review critical scientific data and address questions related to human relevance of experimental data, modes of action, exposure information, dose-response assessment, and the potential for cumulative effects. In its evaluation, the committee will consider the strengths and weaknesses of cumulative assessment approaches. The committee will provide recommendations to EPA on conducting a cumulative risk assessment on phthalate chemicals, including additional research needed. The committee shall consider the applicability of its recommendations for conducting cumulative risk assessment for other chemical classes.

Appendix B

Biographic Information on the Committee on Health Risks of Phthalates

DEBORAH CORY-SLECHTA *(Chair)* is a professor of environmental medicine at the University of Rochester School of Medicine and Dentistry. She was formerly director of the Environmental and Occupational Health Sciences Institute and chair of the Department of Environmental and Occupational Medicine at the University of Medicine and Dentistry of New Jersey, Robert Wood Johnson Medical School. Her research interests include the relationships between neurotransmitter systems and behavior and how such relationships are altered by exposure to environmental toxicants, particularly the role of environmental neurotoxicants in developmental disabilities and neurodegenerative diseases. Dr. Cory-Slechta has served on numerous national research review and advisory panels, including those for the National Institutes of Health, the Environmental Protection Agency, and the Centers for Disease Control and Prevention. She served on the National Research Council's Committee on Human Health Risks of Trichloroethylene and the Committee on Toxicology and on the Institute of Medicine's Committee on Gulf War and Health: Literature Review of Pesticides and Solvents. She received her PhD from the University of Minnesota.

EDMUND CROUCH is a senior scientist with Cambridge Environmental, Inc. He has published widely on environmental quality, biostatistics, risk assessment, and presentation and analysis of uncertainties. He is a coauthor of a major text on risk assessment, *Risk/Benefit Analysis*. Dr. Crouch serves as an expert adviser to various local and national agencies concerned with public health and the environment and has served on nine National Research Council committees. He has written computer programs for the sophisticated analysis of results of carcinogenesis bioassays, has developed algorithms (on the levels of both theory and computer implementation) for the objective quantification of waste-site contamination, and has designed Monte Carlo simulations for the characterization of uncertainties and variabilities inherent in health risk assessment. He received his PhD from the University of Cambridge, England, in high-energy physics.

PAUL FOSTER is the acting chief of the Toxicology Operations Branch and deputy director of the National Toxicology Program's Center for the Evaluation of Risks to Human Reproduction at the National Institute of Environmental Health Sciences (NIEHS) in Research Triangle Park, NC. His recent research has focused on the mechanisms of environmental chemical and drug effects on reproductive development. Before joining NIEHS in 2002, he was the director of the research program in endocrine, reproductive, and developmental toxicology at the CIIT Centers for Health Research. Dr. Foster's research interests include the potential human health effects of environmental endocrine disruptors (particularly antiandrogens), mechanisms of testicular toxicity, early testicular Leydig cell dysfunction induced by chemicals as a prelude to hyperplasia and tumors, and the toxicokinetic and dynamic characteristics of the induction of reproductive and developmental toxicity. He also has a broad interest in risk-assessment issues in those subjects. Dr. Foster has served on numerous national and international advisory committees dealing with reproductive toxicology and endocrine disruption, including the Federal Advisory Committee on the Environmental Protection Agency's Endocrine Disruptor Screening Program. He has served on National Research Council committees, including the Subcommittee on Reproductive and Developmental Toxicology. He earned a PhD in biochemistry and toxicology at Brunel University, United Kingdom.

MARY FOX is assistant professor in the Department of Health Policy and Management at the Johns Hopkins Bloomberg School of Public Health. Her research is focused on developing cumulative risk assessment to inform public-health decision-making. Dr. Fox has applied cumulative-risk methods in numerous community health assessments. Her current research is directed at national-level decision-making and includes the relationship between exposure to a mixture of nephrotoxic metals and renal function and model uncertainty and the potential for error in cumulative exposure assessments for pesticides as mandated by the Food Quality Protection Act. Dr. Fox earned her MPH from the University of Rochester School of Medicine and Dentistry and her PhD from the Johns Hopkins Bloomberg School of Public Health.

KEVIN GAIDO is senior investigator with the Hamner Institutes for Health Sciences. His research specialty is receptor-mediated mechanisms of toxicity. Dr. Gaido's current interests focus on chemical interactions with steroid-hormone receptors and the resulting cellular and molecular responses. Dr. Gaido earned his PhD in pharmacology and toxicology from the West Virginia University Medical Center.

MAIDA GALVEZ is an assistant professor in the Department of Community and Preventive Medicine and the Department of Pediatrics at the Mount Sinai

School of Medicine. She is a board-certified pediatrician who directs Mount Sinai's Pediatric Environmental Health Specialty Unit and practices general pediatrics. She is co-principal investigator and a designated new investigator of a research project funded by the National Institute of Environmental Health Sciences (NIEHS) and the Environmental Protection Agency, "Growing Up Healthy in East Harlem," a community-based participatory research project examining the environmental determinants of childhood obesity. She is also coinvestigator of a project funded by NIEHS and the National Cancer Institute to assess environmental determinants of puberty in girls. Her research interests include the urban built environment, endocrine disruptors, and childhood growth and development. Dr. Galvez earned her MD and MPH from the Mount Sinai School of Medicine.

CHRIS GENNINGS is professor of biostatistics at the Virginia Commonwealth University and the director of the research incubator for the Center for Clinical and Translational Research. Her research interests include nonlinear regression modeling, categorical data analysis, analysis of complex mixtures, and statistical issues in mixture toxicology, and she has published extensively on these topics. She has a research project on empirical approaches for evaluating sufficiently similar complex mixtures and is the director of a training grant focused on the integration of mixture toxicology, toxicogenomics, and statistics. She earned her PhD in biostatistics from the Virginia Commonwealth University.

J. PAUL GILMAN is senior vice president and chief sustainability officer for Convanta Energy. Previously, he served as director of the Oak Ridge Center for Advanced Studies and as assistant administrator for research and development in the Environmental Protection Agency. He also worked in the Office of Management and Budget, where he had oversight responsibilities for the Department of Energy (DOE) and all other science agencies, and in DOE, where he advised the secretary of energy on scientific and technical matters. From 1993 to 1998, Dr. Gilman was the executive director of the Commission on Life Sciences and the Board on Agriculture and Natural Resources of the National Research Council. He is a member of the National Research Council Board on Environmental Studies and Toxicology. Dr. Gilman earned PhDs in ecology and evolutionary biology from Johns Hopkins University.

RUSS HAUSER is professor of environmental and occupational epidemiology in the Departments of Environmental Health and Epidemiology of the Harvard School of Public Health. His research focuses on the effects of environmental and occupational chemicals on reproductive health with emphasis on fertility and pregnancy outcomes. He is conducting epidemiologic studies on the relationship of chlorinated chemicals, pesticides, bisphenol A, and phthalates with male and female reproductive health. He is also conducting a prospective cohort study on children in Chapaevsk, Russia, where he is investigating the relationship of exposure to dioxins and dioxin-like compounds with growth and pubertal development. He recently began a two-state study in collaboration with researchers from Yale University on genetic and environmental risk factors for testicular germ-cell cancer. He has served on two Institute of Medicine Committees on Gulf War and Health and the National Research Council Committee on the Review of the National Children's Study Research Plan. He is an associate editor and on the Advisory Board of *Environmental Health Perspectives* and on the Editorial Boards of the *Journal of Exposure Science* and *Environmental Epidemiology*. He is chair-elect of the recently established Environment and Reproduction Special Interest Group of the American Society for Reproductive Medicine. He received an MD from Albert Einstein College of Medicine and an MPH and ScD from the Harvard School of Public Health, where he completed a residency in occupational medicine. He is board-certified in occupational medicine.

ANDREAS KORTENKAMP is professor and head of the Centre for Toxicology at the University of London, School of Pharmacy. His research focuses on the effects of multicomponent mixtures of endocrine-active chemicals. The thrust of his work is to assess whether the effects of mixtures of chemicals can be predicted quantitatively on the basis of information on their individual potencies. Dr. Kortenkamp's research interests lie in environmental pollutants that have the potential to cause cancer. For some years, he has concentrated on endocrine-active chemicals in the environment and their potential role in the rising incidences of breast cancer and testicular cancer. His earlier work was on the mode of action of chromium (VI) compounds, which are recognized occupational carcinogens. Dr. Kortenkamp earned his PhD from Bremen University, Germany.

JEFFREY PETERS is professor of molecular toxicology at the Pennsylvania State University. His research interests include the roles of the peroxisome-proliferator-activated receptors (PPARs) in the regulation of homeostasis, toxicity, and carcinogenesis with extensive application of null mouse models. The goal of his research is to identify functional roles of the PPARs in the etiology and prevention of carcinogenesis. Dr. Peters is also conducting research to delineate the role of the PPARs in the regulation of homeostasis, including body composition, tissue-specific gene expression, serum lipid biochemistry, and atherosclerosis. Results of the research will determine mechanisms that regulate physiologic lipid metabolism by using different activators reported to interact through PPARs. He earned a PhD in nutrition science from the University of California, Davis.

DONNA VORHEES is a principal scientist with the Science Collaborative, where she consults on human health risk assessment for a variety of municipal, federal, and industrial clients. She is also an adjunct assistant professor at the Boston University School of Public Health, where she teaches a course in risk-assessment methods. She has extensive experience in addressing environmental questions arising from multipathway human exposure to chemicals that have been released to indoor and outdoor environments at federal and state hazardous-waste sites. Her research interests include development of probabilistic human exposure models, field surveys to collect data needed to support risk assessment, identification of research priorities for improving dredged-material management, and preparation of environmental-health educational materials. Dr. Vorhees conducted probabilistic analyses of multipathway exposure to polychlorinated biphenyls (PCBs) in residences near the New Bedford Harbor, MA, Superfund site, to PCBs and pesticides that accumulate in fish from an offshore dredged-material disposal site, and to PCBs, dioxins, and furans that accumulate in agricultural products from the floodplain of a contaminated river. She is an active member of the Society for Risk Analysis and the International Society of Exposure Analysis and served on the National Research Council Committee on Sediment Dredging at Superfund Megasites. Dr. Vorhees earned her ScD in environmental health from the Harvard School of Public Health.

MARY SNOW WOLFF is professor of community and preventive medicine and professor of oncologic sciences at the Mount Sinai School of Medicine. She is also director of the Center for Children's Environmental Health and Disease Prevention Research, a multidisciplinary research program funded by the National Institutes of Health and the Environmental Protection Agency. Her research interests center around application of biologic markers to determine exposures of humans to chemicals that occur in the environment. Environmental exposures are considered in the context of diet, lifestyle, and individual susceptibility factors and in the context of their relationship to cancer risk, to reproductive dysfunction, and to developmental disorders. She has been involved in numerous studies of occupational and ambient environmental exposures to polycyclic aromatic hydrocarbons, organochlorine pesticides, and polychlorinated biphenyls. She has also investigated lead poisoning, dermal exposures, and chemicals in breast milk. She has collaborated in several studies of breast-cancer risk associated with environmental exposures and the genetic determinants of the risk. More recently, she has shifted emphasis to newly identified exposures that may be most relevant to the 21st century. Dr. Wolff earned a PhD in organic chemistry from Yale University.

Appendix C

Analysis of a Mixture of Five Phthalates: A Case Study

The objective of this appendix is to provide details on an approach to the evaluation of "low-dose" mixture effects (see discussion in Chapter 5) by using data on a mixture of phthalates. There are many ways of conceptualizing a critical dose of each chemical in a mixture associated with "no observable effect," such as no-observed-adverse-effect levels (NOAELs) or benchmark doses (BMDs). For illustration purposes, a BMD associated with a benchmark response (BMR) of 5% is estimated for each chemical in a mixture of phthalates and is used to determine a "mixture BMD" for a specified mixing ratio, assuming dose addition. The choice of a 5% BMR is for illustration only; other values may be selected. The mixture BMD depends on the mixing ratio of the components, and a tiered analysis strategy is described to determine critical doses of the chemicals in the mixture.

Howdeshell et al. (2008) reported on the effect that a mixture of five phthalate esters (BBP, DBP, DEHP, DIBP, and DPP) had on fetal testicular testosterone production. The mixture was selected so that the dose of each phthalate was proportional to a dose that yielded about equal reduction in testosterone when the components were given alone; that is, they used BBP, DBP, DEHP, and DIBP each at one dose and DPP at one-third that dose. Single-chemical data were used to predict the effect of the mixture at the specified ratio assuming dose addition; the observed fixed-ratio mixture dose-response data were compared with the dose-response predicted under dose addition. However, Howdeshell et al. did not use the dose-addition formula given in Chapter 4 (Equation 1) but rather an approximate approach to dose addition that used the average of the Hill slopes for the individual chemicals. The analytic method used in this appendix is based on a more general dose-additive model than and a somewhat different dose-response model from that used by Howdeshell et al. (2008). Here, dose addition is performed by using the formula from Chapter 4 (Equation 1) with the different slopes of the dose-response curves of the mixture components, and equality of the slopes is tested. Specifically, a nonlinear logistic dose-response model is used to facilitate a point estimate of a BMD—corresponding to a BMR of 5%—for each chemical alone. A mixture BMD is estimated from the dose-additive model and compared with that estimated from the observed mixture data at the specified mixing ratio. Furthermore, the dose-additive model is used to demonstrate that the mixture BMD is not constant across mixing ratios. That is, the point estimate of the mixture BMD predicted under dose addition is shown to be numerically different if observed and hypothetical mixing ratios of the five chemicals are used. The illustration is concluded with a description of a tiered analytic strategy for mixtures.

METHODS

Data were kindly provided by Earl Gray, Jr., in the Reproductive Toxicology Division, National Health and Environmental Effects Research Laboratory, Office of Research and Development, Environmental Protection Agency, Research Triangle Park, NC.

Experimental Data. Pregnant Sprague-Dawley rats were dosed by gavage on gestation day (GD) 8-18 with either vehicle control (dose, 0), a dose of one of the chemicals, or a dose of the mixture of five phthalates (BBP, DBP, DEHP, DIBP, and DPP) in a mixing ratio of 3:3:3:3:1. DEP was also evaluated in the single-chemical studies but showed no effect; the DEP data have been retained because they provide additional information on variability. Both single-chemical and mixture studies were conducted in blocks (incomplete block design) with one or two dams per treatment per block with two to four blocks per chemical for a total of 166 litters across chemicals and doses. Testosterone was extracted on GD 18 from the testes of the first three males in each litter and measured with radioimmunoassay. Details are given in Howdeshell et al. (2008). The average of the two measurements (one per testis) for each fetus was used in the analysis herein.

Initial Statistical Analysis. A mixed-effects analysis of variance was used to test for differences in control-group means while adjusting for intralitter correlated data. There was a significant difference in the control-group means of testosterone (in nanograms per milliliter of medium) between studies and a significant block effect, so the data from all studies were adjusted by the average control-group value per block (giving percent of control).

Construction of an Additivity Model. The general strategy for the analysis of the data was to use the single-chemical data to fit a nonlinear logistic model of the mean (μ) testosterone concentration (percent of control) for the five single chemicals and for the fixed-ratio mixture (in terms of total dose), that is,

$$\mu_i = \alpha_i + \frac{(1-\alpha_i)[1+\exp(-\beta_{0i})]}{1+\exp[-(\beta_{0i}+\beta_i x)]},$$

where x is the dose, α_i is the parameter associated with the maximum effect for the ith chemical or mixture, β_i is the (negative) parameter associated with the slope for the ith chemical or mixture, and β_{0i} is the parameter associated with the shape of the curve. The term $[1+\exp(-\beta_{0i})]$ was included in the numerator to force the mean to equal 1 for the control group ($x = 0$). It was assumed that the observed relative testosterone concentration differed from the model mean, μ, by additive independent zero-mean normally distributed random terms representing between-pup (within-litter) and between-litter variations (that is, a nonlinear mixed-effects model was used with a linear random-effect, adjusting for intraliter correlations). Preliminary analyses demonstrated that the sample variances among chemicals, doses, and litters increased with the sample means; this suggested that the within-litter variation is proportional to the mean. When the within-litter values were adjusted for the dose-group mean, the variation was relatively similar and suggested a common interlitter variance. The model adopted therefore set the within-litter variance to be proportional to the predicted mean and set the between-litter standard deviation to be constant. The model was estimated with all three parameters per chemical and mixture (18 mean parameters and two parameters for the standard deviations).

When the model dose-response curve is inverted, the dose, $ED_i(\mu_0)$, of the ith chemical that is required to produce a given mean, μ_0, is

$$ED_i(\mu_0) = \frac{\ln\left[\dfrac{(\mu_0-\alpha_i)}{1-\mu_0+(1-\alpha_i)\exp(-\beta_{0i})}\right]-\beta_{0i}}{\beta_i}.$$

Therefore, if component doses of a mixture are given by $a_i t_{add}$, where the a_i are fixed proportions and t_{add} is the total mixture dose, then the general dose-additive model (see Altenburger et al. 2000 and Gennings et al. 2004) gives the dose-response curve for this fixed-proportion mixture as

$$t_{add} = \left[\sum_{i=1}^{5}\frac{a_i}{ED_i(\mu_0)}\right]^{-1}$$

$$= \left[\sum_{i=1}^{5}\frac{a_i}{\dfrac{\ln\left[\dfrac{(\mu_0-\alpha_i)}{1-\mu_0+(1-\alpha_i)\exp(-\beta_{0i})}\right]-\beta_{0i}}{\beta_i}}\right]^{-1}.$$

The mixture data were also fitted to a nonlinear model of the same form, in terms of total dose, as used for the components. The mixture BMD with a 5% BMR was estimated from the mixture model and from the dose-additive model.[1]

For comparison, an independent-action model based on percentage of response to individual chemicals (π_i) was estimated, where[2]

$$\pi_i = \frac{\mu_i - \alpha_i}{1 - \alpha_i} = \frac{1 + \exp(-\beta_{0i})}{1 + \exp\left[-\left(\beta_{0i} + \beta_i x\right)\right]}.$$

If π measures the fraction of the maximum response, then

$$\pi_{ind} = \prod_{i=1}^{5} \pi_i.$$

It is important to note that the independent-action model as used here is not a probabilistic model; it makes the conceptual leap of substituting fractional effect (the fraction of the maximum response) for probability of occurrence (see Chapter 4). It is not based on the assumption of statistical independence. Moreover, there is no way to estimate the maximum effect by using independent action; here, for illustration, it is assumed that the maximum effect is 100% suppression of testosterone because the maximum likelihood estimate for DEHP alone has a maximum effect of 100% suppression.

RESULTS

Preliminary analyses indicated significant differences in mean testosterone concentrations among the vehicle control groups and a significant difference in the means among the blocks within control groups. Therefore, the later analyses were based on percent control values, which were calculated by dividing the average testosterone concentration per pup by the corresponding intrablock average control mean.

The nonlinear logistic mixed-effects model was fitted to the dose-response data from each single chemical and to the mixture data in terms of total dose; the model allowed intralitter correlated data. All five slope parameters were negative and significant, indicating that as the dose increases, there is a significant decrease in testosterone concentration. The five slope parameters were statisti-

---

[1]The model parameters were estimated by maximizing the likelihood of the observations, and confidence limits were estimated with the profile likelihood method. All calculations were performed in an Excel spreadsheet with components coded in Visual Basic for Applications.

[2]Recall that *response* in this case is the reduction in testosterone concentration and that there is a maximum response.

cally inhomogeneous (p = 0.03, likelihood ratio test) with point estimates ranging from −0.002 to −0.040 per milligram per kilogram per day. Figure C-1 provides the observations and model-predicted dose-response curves (for the mean response, at the maximum likelihood) for the five phthalates. In general, the data are adequately represented by the nonlinear logistic model. Figure C-2 presents the observed mixture data in terms of total dose. The solid curve is the model fit based on the nonlinear logistic model, which adequately represents the observed data. The dashed curve (Figure C-2A) is the dose-response model for the mixture under the assumption of additivity. For comparison, the predicted independent-action dose-response curve is provided in Figure C-2B. In this case, the experimentally observed mixture data are adequately approximated by both the dose-additive model and the independent-action model. In most cases, mixture data are not available to make such a comparison, and single-chemical data are used to approximate the mixture through an additivity model; in this case, dose addition is a reasonable default to use when mixture data are not available.

It is of interest to determine a critical dose for the mixture of five phthalates and compare the adjusted critical doses of the individual components with their unadjusted critical doses. When the mixing ratio of the chemicals is specified, a BMD can be estimated for the mixture by using dose addition. BMD estimates for each of the five chemicals are provided in Table C-1 with lower one-sided 95% confidence limits. BMDs for the mixture (with a specified mixing ratio) and as predicted under additivity for the same mixing ratio (with the proportion of the ith chemical denoted by a_i) were estimated with the single-chemical and mixture models (Table C-1). Specifically, the BMD for the mixture (with fixed mixing ratio) under additivity is estimated as

$$t_{add} = \left(\sum_{i=1}^{5} \frac{a_i}{BMD_i} \right)^{-1} = \left(\frac{0.23}{116} + \frac{0.23}{30} + \frac{0.23}{49} + \frac{0.08}{25} + \frac{0.23}{126} \right)^{-1} = 52 \text{ mg/kg-d.}$$

The mixture BMD as predicted by dose addition depends on the mixing ratios of the chemicals. To illustrate that point, consider three mixing ratios of the five phthalates for which single-chemical data are available (from the study by Howdeshell et al. 2008). Table C-2 includes the mixing proportions for each case and the corresponding concentrations of each chemical in such mixtures at the mixture BMD (assuming dose addition). Such mixture BMDs depend on the mixing ratio of the chemicals. A tiered analytic strategy is suggested by consideration of the following and other cases.

• Case 1 is based on a mixture in which the mixing ratio for each single-chemical component concentration is proportional to the BMD for each single chemical. The single-chemical component concentrations in the BMD mixture correspond to dividing each BMD by the number of active chemicals in the mixture—here, five. The single-chemical component concentrations in the BMD mixture can be considered as adjusted critical values—any mixture that contains single-chemical component concentrations that are each less than or equal to their adjusted critical values[3] will (under dose addition) invoke a response less than the BMR. In case 1, the mixture BMD is 69 mg/kg-d under additivity, and the adjusted critical values for the five chemicals range from 5 mg/kg-d for DPP to 25 mg/kg-d for DIBP (Table C-2). This case is especially simple because the adjusted critical values are just one-fifth of the single-chemical BMDs (Table C-1). When the exposure concentration of each single chemical in some mixture is below the adjusted critical value (for *any* mixing ratio), the response to the mixture is associated with a lower BMR than that used to construct the adjusted critical values (here, the BMR is 5%).

• Cases 2 and 3 are based on exposure data presented in Table 2-2; data on DPP as a parent compound were not included, and it is omitted from these two cases. Table 2-2 presents urinary concentrations of metabolites of the parent compounds, but the fraction of the parent diester that ends up in the urine varies widely among the phthalates. For example, 5-10% of DEHP is excreted as

TABLE C-1 Estimated BMDs Associated with 5% BMR[a] for Single Chemicals and Mixture Data Based on Nonlinear Logistic Model and Estimated with Mixed-Effects Model Accounting for Intralitter Correlated Data[b]

Chemical	BMD (mg/kg-d)	Lower One-Sided 95% Confidence Limit (mg/kg-d)
BBP	116	66
DBP	30	20
DEHP	49	31
DPP	25	10
DIBP	126	47
Mixture	74	39
Mixture (additivity)	52	39

[a]The response evaluated here is the fractional reduction of testosterone concentration relative to the testosterone concentration at zero dose. Other definitions could be contemplated, such as the change relative to the maximum reduction achievable or, in view of the variation observed in average testosterone concentrations at zero dose between different groups of animals, some change related to a measure of the width of the distribution of those zero-dose testosterone concentrations. The choice here has been arbitrarily selected for demonstration purposes.
[b]The mixture components are each at 23% except DPP, which is 8% of the mixture. Study details are included in Howdeshell et al. (2008).

---

[3]Any particular set of adjusted critical values have to be treated together as a set for a particular mixing ratio of the components. There must be no mixing and matching of adjusted critical values obtained from different mixtures.

TABLE C-2 Three Mixtures to Illustrate an Approach to Calculating Adjusted Critical Doses for Single Chemicals in a Mixture[a]

	Mixing Ratios That Sum to 1 (Single-Chemical Dose [mg/kg] in Mixture BMD, Assuming Additivity)[b]					Mixture BMD, Assuming Additivity (mg/kg)
	BBP	DBP	DEHP	DPP	DIBP	
Case	a_1	a_2	a_3	a_5	a_6	t_{add}
1	0.336	0.086	0.143	0.072	0.363	
	(23.3)	(6.0)	(9.9)	(5.0)	(25.2)	**69.3**
2	0.13	0.19	0.66		0.02	
	(6.2)	(9.0)	(31.4)	—	(1.0)	**47.6**
3	0.02	0.38	0.48		0.12	
	(0.8)	(16.1)	(20.3)	—	(5.1)	**42.4**

[a]Case 1 corresponds to dividing each single chemical BMD by 5 (the number of active chemicals in the mixture). Case 2 is based on the relative proportion of the parent compound from its metabolites at the 50th percentile as evaluated in the NHANES study for the five chemicals (see Table 2-2). Case 3 is based on the relative proportion of the parent compound from its metabolites at the 50th percentile as evaluated in the Wittassek et al. (2007) study (see Table 2-2). The mixture BMD depends on the mixing ratio.
[b]The single-chemical doses for the mixture BMD under additivity sum to the mixture BMD in the last column.

MEHP, whereas more than 90% of DBP is excreted as MBP. For this example, we assumed that the sum of MEHP, MECPP, MEOHP, and MEHHP (DEHP metabolites) represents 50% of parent DEHP. Because less is known about the excretion of BBP, DBP, and DIBP as measured by the listed metabolites, we assumed that the excretion of the corresponding metabolites is roughly similar to the exposure to the parent compound. So, for illustration only, the mixing proportions of the four parent compounds were calculated on the basis of the proportion of the sum across the metabolites (using the 50th percentile values) for the four parent compounds, with the DEHP metabolites doubled. Case 2 corresponds to the values from the National Health and Nutrition Examination Survey (NHANES); case 3 corresponds to the German study values (see Table 2-2). For case 2, the mixture BMD is 48 mg/kg under dose addition, and the adjusted critical values for the remaining four chemicals range from 1 mg/kg for DIBP to 31 mg/kg for DEHP (Table C-2). For case 3, the mixture BMD is 42 mg/kg under additivity, and the adjusted critical values for the remaining four chemicals range from 1 mg/kg for BBP to 20 mg/kg for DEHP (Table C-2).

In contrast with the evaluation of single chemicals, the critical dose (here, 69, 48, and 42 mg/kg for the three cases considered) of a mixture and the adjusted critical values for the components clearly depend on the mixing ratio.

How should adjusted critical doses be specified for individual chemicals in a mixture when exposure information is not available (that is, the doses and mixing ratios of the chemicals in the mixture are not known or are not constant)? The committee suggests that a tiered approach be considered.

- First, determine whether the single-chemical doses in the exposure of concern are all below the adjusted critical value specified by dividing the critical values (here, the BMD associated with a fixed BMR) of the single chemicals by the number of active chemicals in the mixture (case 1 in Table C-2). If so, the response to the mixture is less than the BMR, assuming general dose addition. There is no need to go any further.
- Second, if one or more of the single-chemical doses in the exposure of concern exceeds the adjusted critical value specified for the mixture in step 1, determine the mixing ratio of the exposure of concern and recalculate the critical dose for the specific mixture ratio (for example, cases 2 and 3 in Table C-2). If all single-chemical exposures are below the adjusted critical doses for the mixture of concern, the response to the mixture is less than the BMR, assuming general dose addition.

In Table C-2 for cases 2 and 3, assumptions would be made to determine doses of a parent compound on the basis of metabolite concentrations. If, for example, the calculated dose of DEHP exceeds 10 mg/kg (from case 1), a more refined estimate of an adjusted critical dose could be based on the mixing ratios obtained from exposure estimates (case 2 or 3). That is, the exposure to DEHP may be increased if exposures to other chemicals are lower than considered in case 1. If the exposure to each chemical is below the single-chemical adjusted critical value for the specified mixture ratio (case 2 or 3), the response could be claimed to be less than the selected BMR.

DISCUSSION

The additivity model described here was based on a nonlinear logistic model with the potential for a maximum effect other than zero testosterone. Howdeshell et al. (2008) used the nonlinear Hill model, assuming that the maximum effect was complete suppression of testosterone, and approximated the dose-addition procedure by using an average Hill slope for the mixture. The analyses of each model included similar figures (Figure C-2 here; Figure 2B in Howdeshell et al. 2008) that compared the mixture data, the nonlinear model fit to mixture data, and the model predicted by dose addition. Both showed that the dose-additive model fell below the mixture model. Howdeshell et al. did not make a statistical comparison of the two models; they claimed that a dose-additive relationship adequately represented the data. As seen in Figure C-2, the dose-additive model used here is similar to the observed mixture model; a formal statistical comparison of the two curves was not conducted.

The point of the analysis illustrated here was to determine a mixture BMD by using dose addition and to show that its value depends on the mixing ratio.

That required an estimation of a BMD for each component in the mixture; a nonlinear logistic model was used here for illustration. A comparison of the results that would be obtained with other models was not conducted. The development and dissemination of methods that result in inference that does not depend on a specific model constitute an important field of research. Bayesian approaches have been suggested in which the resulting inferences include the uncertainty associated with model selection, as well as parameter uncertainty.

In accordance with the discussion in Chapter 5, the evaluation of critical doses in this illustration was based on BMDs. Nyribihizi et al. (2008) compare BMDs for experimentally observed mixture data with a fixed mixing ratio and the corresponding BMD under additivity. Their approach is similar to that used here. Other approaches, such as the use of NOAELs, are possible; the limitations of the use of NOAELs have been discussed extensively (see, for example, EPA 2000).

The illustration in this appendix included the use of approximate mixing ratios of the chemicals estimated from urinary concentrations. Such estimates required many simplifying assumptions. The availability of the supporting data relating urinary metabolites and parent compound exposure concentrations varies among the chemicals. Exposures probably differ between infants, children, and adults—a variation not considered in our calculations. However, the approach is generic and can be repeated for different mixing ratios to account for observed exposures.

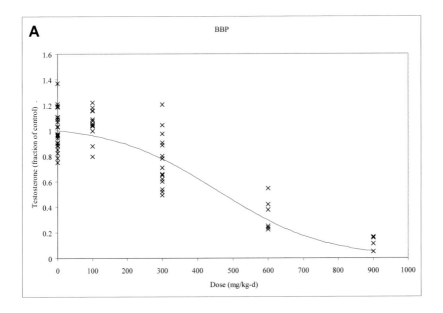

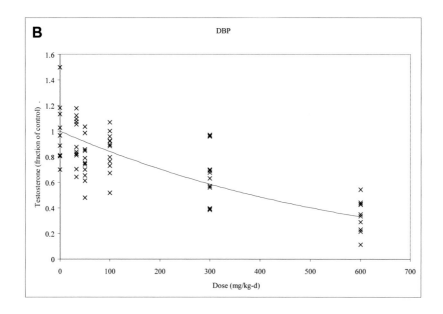

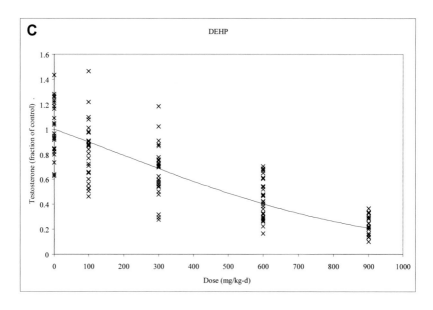

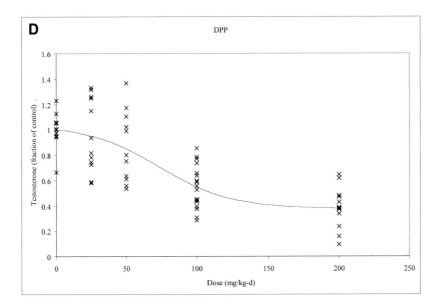

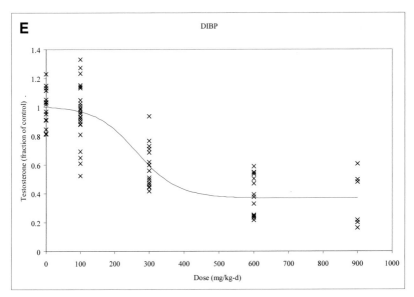

FIGURE C-1 Average testosterone concentration (as percent of control) per pup (*) vs dose of five single chemicals with maximum likelihood dose-response curves used in additivity model.

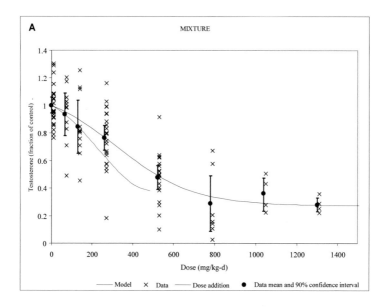

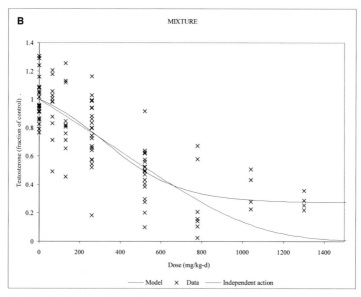

FIGURE C-2 (A) Observed (*) and model-predicted dose-response curves for mixture of five phthalates based on the nonlinear logistic model for the mixture data (solid curve) and as predicted under additivity (dashed curve). The mixing ratio of the five phthalates was 3:3:3:3:1 for BBP, DBP, DEHP, DIBP, and DPP, that is, 0.23, 0.23, 0.23, 0.23, and 0.08 of the mixture. (B) For comparison, the prediction using an independent-action model based on percentage of response.

REFERENCES

Altenburger, R., T. Backhaus, W. Boedeker, M. Faust, M. Scholze, and L.H. Grimme. 2000. Predictability of the toxicity of multiple chemical mixtures to *Vibrio fischeri:* Mixtures composed of similarly acting chemicals. Environ. Toxicol. Chem. 19(9):2341-2347.

EPA (U.S. Environmental Protection Agency). 2000. Benchmark Dose Technical Guidance Document. External Review Draft. EPA/630/R-00/001. Risk Assessment Forum, U.S. Environmental Protection Agency, Washington, DC [online]. Available: http://www.epa.gov/ncea/pdfs/bmds/BMD-External_10_13_2000.pdf [accessed July 25, 2008].

Gennings, C., W.H. Carter, Jr., E.W. Carney, G.D. Charles, B.B. Gollapudi, and R.A. Carchman. 2004. A novel flexible approach for evaluating fixed ratio mixtures of full and partial agonists. Toxicol. Sci. 80(1):134-150.

Howdeshell, K.L., V.S. Wilson, J. Furr, C.R. Lambright, C.V. Rider, C.R. Blystone, A.K. Hotchkiss, and L.E. Gray, Jr. 2008. A mixture of five phthalate esters inhibits fetal testicular testosterone production in the Sprague-Dawley rat in a cumulative, dose-additive manner. Toxicol. Sci. 105(1):153-165.

Nyirabahizi, E., C. Gennings, W.W. Piegorsch, S. Yeatts, M.J. DeVito, and K.M. Crofton. 2008. Benchmark doses for chemical mixtures: Evaluation of a mixture of 18 PHAHs. Toxicologist 102(S-1):242 [Abstract No. 1177].

Wittassek, M., G.A. Wiesmuller, H.M. Koch, R. Eckard, L. Dobler, J. Muller, J. Angerer, and C. Schluter. 2007. Internal phthalate exposure over the last two decades—a retrospective human biomonitoring study. Int. J. Hyg. Environ. Health 210(3-4):319-333.

Appendix D

Evaluating Multiple End Points Simultaneously in a Mixture of Three Antiandrogens: A Case Study

An important step in risk assessment is the selection of end points for analysis. For single-chemical risk assessment, the most sensitive end point has often served as the basis of evaluation, although current guidance suggests a more nuanced approach (EPA 2002, 2005). Some authors have considered models that combine multiple end points in the same model and therefore avoid having to select the most sensitive end point. For example, Sammel et al. (1997) used a latent-variable model for mixed discrete and continuous correlated outcomes in which the posterior estimate of the latent variable may be interpreted as a measure of severity. Other authors have used pseudolikelihood estimation when combining continuous and ordinal outcomes to simplify the numerical challenges of using a joint density (see, for example, Faes et al. 2004). One advantage of pseudolikelihood approaches over conditional models is that estimation of a joint benchmark dose is possible; this lends itself to quantitative risk assessment (Geys et al. 1999, 2001; Regan and Catalano 1999; Faes et al. 2004).

The issue is more complex for risk assessment of chemical mixtures. Although a general kind of risk, such as reproductive or developmental risk, may be clear, different chemicals in the mixture may be associated with different sensitive end points. Furthermore, when data on studies and chemicals are combined, there is no guarantee that the same end points were even measured or that the data are available. Such missing-data concerns may result in numerical difficulties in latent-variable and multivariate models. For those reasons and others, a composite score (see, for example, Moser 1991; McDaniel and Moser 1993; Moser et al. 1995, 1997; Shih et al. 2003; Coffey et al. 2007) that combines multiple end points into a single score may be useful.

The objective of this appendix is to illustrate the development of a composite score in the analysis of the effects of a mixture of three antiandrogens on male differentiation in rats (data from Hass et al. 2007; Metzdorff et al. 2007).

Five end points—anogenital distance (AGD), nipple retention (NR), and three organ weights (weights of the ventral prostate, seminal vesicles, and levator ani/bulbocavernosus muscles [LABC])—are assessed. Owing to the nature of the end points and the timing of their measurement, most pups were evaluated either for AGD and NR or for organ weights. The composite score adjusts for either case. As indicated in this example, the end points combined in the composite score may be different (for example, binary or categorical, count, or continuous or interval variables). The approach used here is based on desirability functions. Desirability functions were first proposed by Harrington (1965) for use in optimizing the quality of a manufactured product that is measured by multiple end points. Harrington's approach is used to find the levels of the factors that optimize the overall quality of the many end points (Derringer and Suich 1980; Derringer 1994). It has been widely adopted in manufacturing and among engineers involved in product optimization is the most popular method for simultaneously analyzing many outcomes (Wu 2005). The method has also been applied to the titration of multiple-drug regimens in medical research (Shih et al. 2003) and in dose-response modeling in toxicology studies (Coffey et al. 2007).

Once a composite scoring method is specified, each animal is represented in the data analysis by a single score regardless of the number of variables measured. Dose-response curves are estimated for each chemical, and an additivity model is estimated. In this study, a fixed-ratio mixture of the three chemicals was also experimentally evaluated. It is of interest to determine whether there is evidence of interaction in the region of the mixing ratio and, even if there is evidence of an interaction, how different the dose-response curve of the mixture is from that predicted by dose addition.

METHODS

Experimental data. Data, generously provided by Ulla Hass, are as described in Hass et al. (2007) and Metzdorff et al. (2007). In short, male sexual differentiation was studied after in utero and postnatal exposures to one or a mixture of three antiandrogens (vinclozolin, flutamide, and procymidone). The mixing ratio of the mixture was based on individual potencies for "causing retention of six nipples in male offspring" (Hass et al. 2007). Test chemicals and mixtures were administered by gavage to time-mated nulliparous, young adult Wistar rats from gestation day 7 to the day before expected birth and on postnatal days 1-16. Changes in AGD and NR in male offspring rats were evaluated. The ventral prostate, seminal vesicles, and LABC of one male per litter were excised and weighed.

Composite score. A composite score was calculated based on the basis of the desirability-function method (see, for example, Harrington 1965; Coffey et al. 2007) for the five end points chosen for analysis. In short, for each variable, a function is selected that transforms the observed response to a unitless score (0-1) based on the appropriateness (or desirability) of the response. The individual scores are then combined into a single composite score by using the geometric mean, and a standard statistical analysis can be performed. This flexible approach can handle multiple types of response variables and may include different desirability functions for each variable. Subjectivity in specifying the functions may be minimized by using consensus expert opinion.

Each of the five variables of interest was transformed to a continuous desirability function, d_i, with values ranging from 0 to 1, where a value of 0 designates the response as not at all desirable, and a value of 1 is assigned to the most desirable response. Although they are not included here, for categorical end points (such as a mild or moderate or severe histopathology score), a value of 0-1 is selected for each category. For continuous end points (such as AGD and NR), the basic shape of the function is determined by whether one is trying to maximize or minimize the response or to aim for a range of target values (see, for example, Shih et al. 2003). For example, a larger AGD value is expected for males, so a "larger is better" shape may be specified by using a logistic function:

$$d_{i(\max)} = \left[1 + \exp\left(-\left(\frac{Y_i - a_i}{b_i} \right) \right) \right]^{-1},$$

where

$$a_i = \frac{Y_{i*} + Y_i^*}{2} \text{ and } b_i = \frac{Y_i^* - Y_{i*}}{2 \ln(\frac{1-\gamma_i}{\gamma_i})}, Y_{i*} < Y_i^*.$$

The parameter a_i is an average of the upper (Y_i^*) and lower (Y_{i*}) bounds of the response being targeted, b_i controls the function spread, and γ_i is defined so that the desirability at Y_{i*} equals γ_i and the desirability at Y_i^* equals $1-\gamma_i$. A minimizing desirability is obtained by reversing the sign of the exponential argument. A target desirability function can then be constructed by multiplying minimizing $(d_{i(\min)})$ and maximizing $(d_{i(\max)})$ desirability functions so that $d_i = d_{i(\max)}{}^* d_{i(\min)}$. The parameters a_i, b_i, and γ_i, allow flexibility in defining the desirability function and the degree of conservativeness to incorporate. The shapes of the individual desirability functions are provided in Figure D-1A-E. The asterisks represent observed data points.

For AGD, a normalized score for the AGD index (Hass et al. 2007) was formed by using "mean AGD indices from unexposed male and female pups" to define the minimum (min) and maximum (max) responses. The normalized score was defined as

$$AGD_{norm} = \frac{AGDindex - min}{max - min}.$$

Thus, a normalized value of 0 represents "complete feminization" and is associated with an undesirable response ($d_i = 0$); a normalized value near 1 represents the average unexposed-male AGD index, a desirable response ($d_i = 1$). The lower 1-percentile of the unexposed males had a normalized value of 0.56 with an interquartile range (IQR) of 0.24. The desirability function was selected so that a normalized value of 0.56 was assigned a score of 0.9; a normalized value of 2IQR below 0.56 (=0.08) was assigned a value of 0.1 (which equals γ in the notation above; see Figure D-1A).

For NR, following Hass et al. (see Hass et al., Table 3), values of 1, 6, and 10 were considered low, medium, and high effects. A desirability function was selected (Figure D-1B) with assigned scores of 0.95, 0.66, and 0.24, respectively. Desirability functions for organ weights (ventral prostate, seminal vesicles, and LABC) in terms of percentage of control were also based on the lower 1-percentile of the unexposed group ($d_i = 0.9$) and 2IQR below the 1-percentile was assigned a value of 0.1 (γ in the notation above). The resulting desirability functions are provided in Figure D-1C-E.

Those individual desirability functions were combined by using the geometric mean to arrive at a composite measure of overall desirability, D, so that

$$D = (d_1 \times d_2 \times ... \times d_k)^{1/k},$$

where k is the number of end points used in the calculation. Although they are not used here, it is also possible to assign different weights to the individual desirability scores:

$$D = (d_1^{w_1} \times d_2^{w_2} \times ... \times d_k^{w_k})^{1/\sum_{j=1}^{k} w_j}.$$

Construction of an additivity model. The general strategy for the analysis of the data was to use the single-chemical data to fit a nonlinear logistic additivity model for the mean composite score, that is,

$$\mu_i = \alpha + \frac{(1-\alpha)}{1 + \exp[-(\beta_0 + \beta_i x)]}$$

for the three single chemicals, where x represents dose.

Following the "single chemical required" method of analysis (see, for example, Casey et al. 2004), the additivity model was used to estimate the dose-response relationship along the fixed-ratio ray of interest (in terms of total dose with mixing ratios a_i) under the hypothesis of additivity:

$$\mu_{add} = \alpha + \frac{(1-\alpha)}{1+\exp[-(\beta_0 + \sum_{i=1}^{c} \beta_i x_i)]}$$

$$= \alpha + \frac{(1-\alpha)}{1+\exp[-(\beta_0 + \sum_{i=1}^{c} \beta_i a_i t)]}$$

$$= \alpha + \frac{(1-\alpha)}{1+\exp[-(\beta_0 + \theta_{add} t)]},$$

where t is total dose and c is the number of chemicals in the mixture (here, 3). The mixture data were also fitted to a nonlinear model in terms of total dose:

$$\mu_{mix} = \alpha + \frac{(1-\alpha)}{1+\exp[-(\beta_0 + \theta_{mix} t)]}.$$

To control for litter effects, the dose-response data were analyzed with a generalized nonlinear mixed-effects model approach with litter as an added random effect. A quasi-Newton iterative algorithm (Proc NLMIXED in SAS; version 9.1) was used for estimation and inference. The test of additivity for the specified mixing ratio is equivalent to testing coincidence between the two models for the mixture. Because the other parameters were assumed to be similar (α and β_0), the hypothesis of coincidence is $H_0 : \theta_{add} = \theta_{mix}$, which can be tested by using a t test with the appropriate variance estimated with the multivariate delta method.

RESULTS

The first step in the analysis is to determine the shapes of desirability curves for each end point under consideration. To illustrate the approach, the summary statistics from the distribution of the unexposed animals (the 1 percentile and the 1 percentile minus 2IQR) were used to establish two points on the curve and thereby specify the shape with a logistic function. The resulting curves are shown in Figure D-1. From the curves, the observed data are transformed into desirability scores of 0-1, where a value of 1 indicates no toxicity and a value of 0 indicates the most severe toxicity. For example (Table D-1), a pup in the highest-dose group of the mixture had an observed AGD index of 6.6, which was transformed to 0.12 in a normalized form. From Figure D-1A, a nor-

TABLE D-1 Demonstration of Calculation of Toxicity Index for Three Rats in Control Group and Two Mixture Dose Groups[a]

End Point	From Control Group (Litter, 1; Block, 1; ID, 5) Observed Response	Desirability Score	From Mixture: Total Dose, 109.19 mg/kg (Litter, 59; Block, 2; ID, 1) Observed Response	Desirability Score	From Mixture: Total Dose, 106.19 mg/kg (Litter, 135; Block, 4; ID, 1) Observed Response	Desirability Score
AGD_BW (Norm_AGD)	10.5 (0.88)	0.99	NR	—	6.6 (0.12)	0.14
Nipples	0	0.97	NR	—	12	0.12
Ventral prostate (%control)	NR	—	0.10	0.43	0.06	0.36
Seminal vesicles (%control)	NR	—	0.30	0.67	0.20	0.56
LABC (%control)	NR	—	0.40	0.80	0.22	0.50
Toxicity index		0.98		0.61		0.27

[a]"Desirability score" can be read from Figure D-1 for observed response values. Observed responses are transformed to %control values for organ weights. Composite score is geometric mean of desirability scores of five end points, adjusted for cases with fewer scores.
NR = not recorded.

malized AGD of 0.12 is associated with a desirability score of 0.14, indicating severe toxicity. For that pup, the calculations of the other four desirability scores followed in a similar manner. The end points demonstrating severe toxicity for the pup were AGD and NR, with scores of 0.14 and 0.12, respectively. The geometric mean of the five values resulted in a toxicity index of 0.27. Calculations are also demonstrated for a pup in the control group and for a pup in a moderate-dose group. In those three rats, the toxicity index decreased as the dose of the mixture increased, indicating that toxicity increased with dose.

Profile plots of the desirability scores of the five end points for each dose group of the mixture study are provided in Figure D-2. Each connected line segment across the end points represents the transformed data from a single pup. The desirability scores transform different end points (one normalized, one count variable, and three expressed in terms of percent control) into a unitless scale of 0-1 that can be compared across end points. The disconnected line segments in the plots illustrate that most pups were either evaluated with AGD and NR or had organ weights measured. In general, the control group and lowest-mixture dose group (7.87 mg/kg) had little indication of toxicity in any of the end points. However, as the dose increased to about 20 mg/kg, there was an indication of worsening NR, AGD was affected at about 40 mg/kg, and organ weights were not highly affected until the dose was about 70 mg/kg. Similar plots are provided in Figure D-4 for each of the single-chemical dose-response studies. The toxicity of the single chemicals was similar to that of the mixture in that NR and AGD were more sensitive than organ weights as specified by the desirability functions.

The composite score was calculated for each pup in the single-chemical and mixture studies by using the geometric mean of the individual desirability scores. The average litter responses across dose are displayed in Figure D-3 as asterisks. There is a clear dose-response relationship for each chemical and for the mixture. The nonlinear logistic model was fitted to these data, and the resulting parameter estimates are provided in Table D-2. In general, the fit of the dose-response curves to each study is adequate (Figure D-3). The maximal-effect parameter (α in Table D-2) for the single chemicals and mixture was estimated as 0.287. All the slope parameters (βs in Table D-2) are negative and significant, indicating that as the dose increases there is an increase in toxicity (a lower value of the composite score).

The additivity model and mixture model were fitted with a common maximal-effect parameter (α) and intercept parameter (β_0), so a test of coincidence between the model for the mixture data and that predicted under additivity from the single-chemical data is a test for a difference in the slope parameters, θ_{mix} and θ_{add} (Table D-2). There is a significant difference in the slopes between

TABLE D-2 Parameter Estimates Based on Nonlinear Logistic Model[a]

Chemical	Parameter	Estimate	Standard Error	p value
	α	0.287	0.015	<0.001
	β_0	3.05	0.151	<0.001
Vinclozolin	β_1	-0.036	0.003	<0.001
Flutamide	β_2	-0.821	0.068	<0.001
Procymidone	β_3	-0.045	0.003	<0.001
	θ_{mix}	-0.086	0.006	<0.001
Additional Estimates				
θ_{add}		-0.055	0.004	<0.001
$\theta_{mix} - \theta_{add}$		-0.031	0.004	<0.001
$ED_{add}(2.5)$		1.67	0.85	0.052
$ED_{mix}(2.5)$		1.06	0.54	0.052
$ED_{add}(2.5) - ED_{mix}(2.5)$		0.60	0.31	0.057

[a]Estimate for scale parameter was 0.02, and variance of random effect due to litter was 0.002, with 95% confidence interval of 0.001-0.003. Estimated dose-response curves are in Figure D-3. Fixed mixing ratios for mixture were $\alpha_1 = 0.62$, $\alpha_2 = 0.02$, and $\alpha_3 = 0.36$ for vinclozolin, flutamide, and procymidone, respectively.

the two models (Table D-2 and Figure D-3D), with the mixture data demonstrating a greater response (a lower composite score) than that predicted under additivity. Although statistically significant, the difference between the two models is most notable in the higher dose range (Figure D-3D). The doses associated with an effect size of 2.5% for the two models are not significantly different (Table D-2).

DISCUSSION

A composite score was developed here for male differentiation for five end points by using a so-called desirability-function method. An advantage of using such a score in evaluation of mixtures is that end points may be combined across studies and chemicals by transforming all end points into a common unitless scale of 0-1. The subjectivity of the initial step of specifying the desirability shapes may be minimized by specifying values on the curves from summary statistics in the control group or by using consensus from subject-matter experts (Coffey et al. 2007). Shih et al. (2003) reported on a simulation study demonstrating a degree of robustness in inference with moderate changes in the shapes of the desirability functions. Furthermore, there is research being conducted to develop methods to optimize desirability-function shapes and their relative importance on the basis of an external empirical measure of severity (Ellis et al. 2008). However, reaching consensus on such issues is not trivial and would require substantial consultation if this method were to be used in a regulatory setting.

When many end points are of interest in evaluating risk posed by exposure to chemical mixtures, multiple statistical tests that may be performed can greatly inflate rates of type I error (concluding that there is an effect when there is none). Multiple comparison adjustments are often too conservative, for example, the Bonferroni correction, which leads to reduced power to detect effects of interest. Thus, use of a composite score focuses the inference to an overall effect and eliminates concern of multiple testing and inflated type I error rates (Coffey et al. 2007).

Hass et al. (2007) reported that the effect of the mixture of three antiandrogens on AGD was predicted "fairly accurately" by dose addition but that the effects on NR "were slightly higher than those expected on the basis of dose addition." Metzdorff et al. (2007) reported that the joint effect of the three antiandrogens on reproductive organ weights was dose-additive. Use of the composite score was driven largely by NR (Figure D-2) and resulted in evidence of a greater effect (lower composite score) of the mixture than that predicted by additivity. Thus, analysis with the composite score was in agreement with the general conclusions reported for the individual end points.

A limitation of the analysis described here is that constant variance among the chemicals and dose groups was assumed. More general assumptions may be more appropriate, as evidenced by plots of the data (Figure D-3). A formal test of equal variance was not conducted. Another limitation of the approach is that the correlation among end points was not accounted for. Wu (2005) describes an extension based on the modified double-exponential desirability function that accounts for correlated multiple characteristics that may be useful in the setting described here.

For general use of composite scores, further evaluation, discussion, and acceptance of the shapes of the desirability functions are necessary. The central motivation is to be able to use a composite score to represent the whole set of common adverse outcomes identified to be of interest for a mixture. For the illustration described in this appendix, the androgen-insufficiency syndrome was evaluated with five end points (AGD, NR, and three reproductive organ weights). The analysis described here is for illustration only; for general use, subject-matter experts would need to achieve some level of acceptance and validation that the composite score did indeed represent the "wholeness" of the syndrome.

A

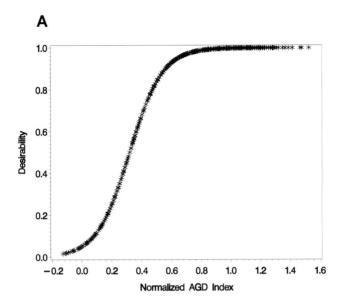

B

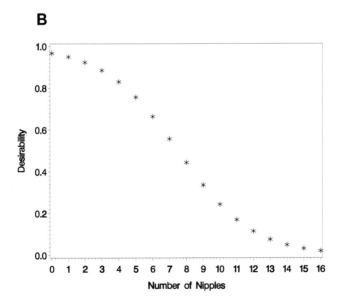

C

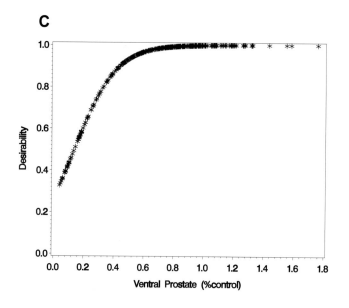

D

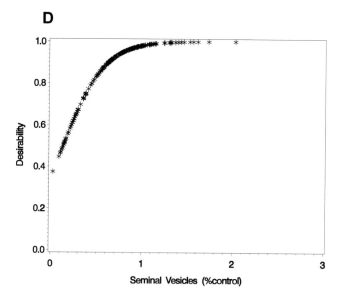

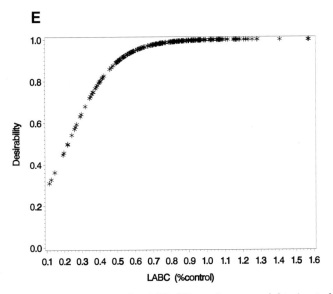

E

FIGURE D-1 Desirability curves for AGD, NR, and organ weights (ventral prostate, seminal vesicle, and LABC). Asterisks represent observed data points.

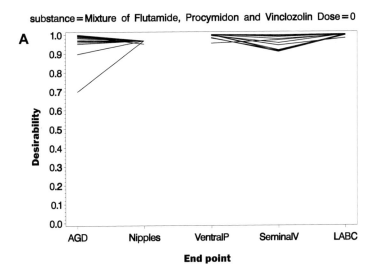

substance = Mixture of Flutamide, Procymidon and Vinclozolin Dose = 0

A

substance=Mixture of Flutamide, Procymidon and Vinclozolin Dose=7.87

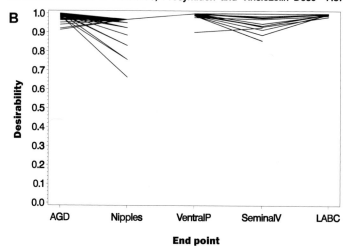

substance=Mixture of Flutamide, Procymidon and Vinclozolin Dose=19.67

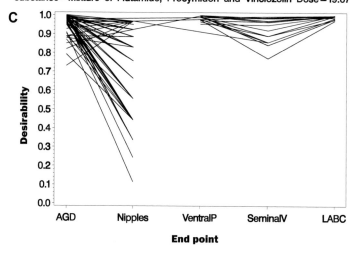

substance = Mixture of Flutamide, Procymidon and Vinclozolin Dose = 39.33

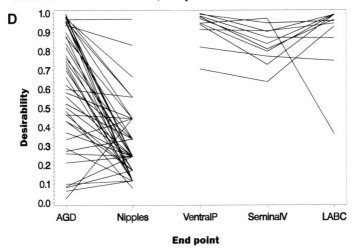

substance = Mixture of Flutamide, Procymidon and Vinclozolin Dose = 70.8

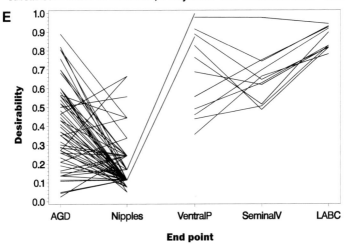

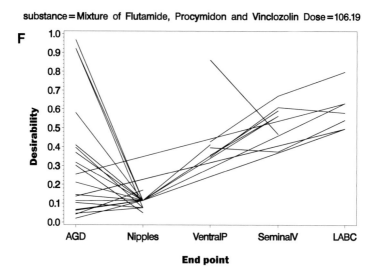

FIGURE D-2 Profile plots for individual pups (connected line segment) in each dose group of mixture data.

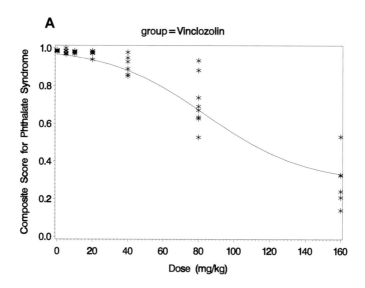

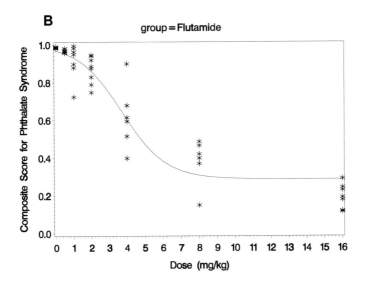

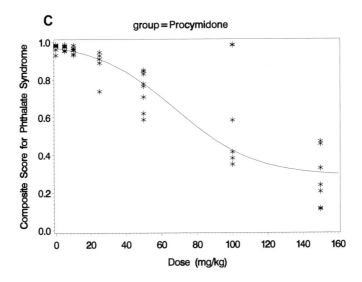

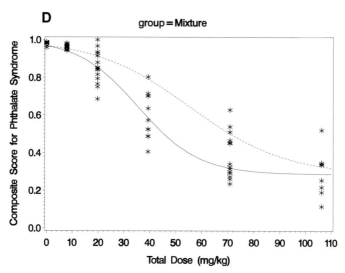

FIGURE D-3 Average calculated toxicity index (composite desirability score) per litter vs dose of three single chemicals and mixture.

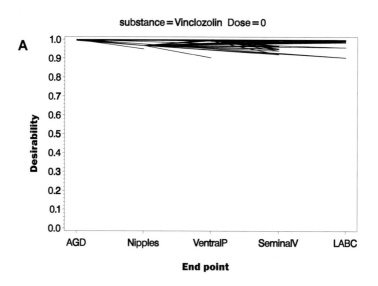

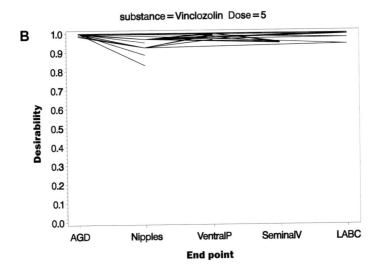

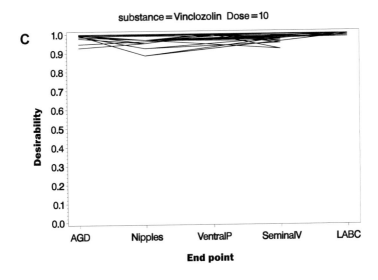

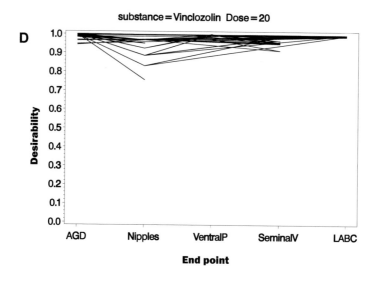

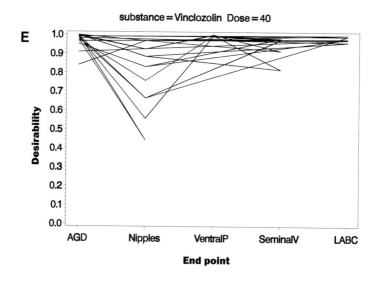

F

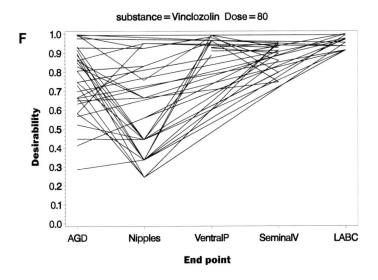

substance = Vinclozolin Dose = 80

G

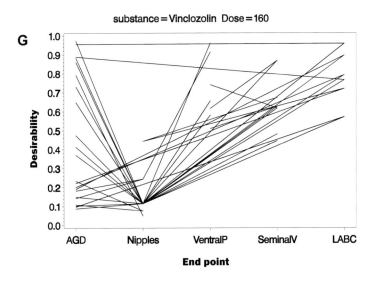

substance = Vinclozolin Dose = 160

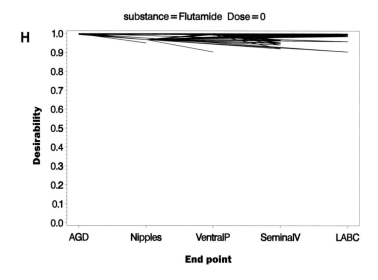

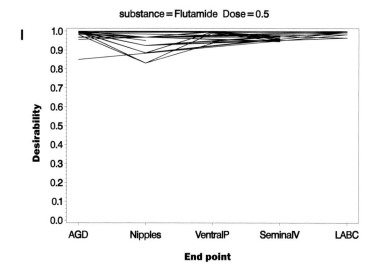

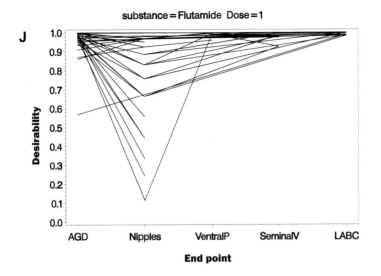

substance = Flutamide Dose = 1

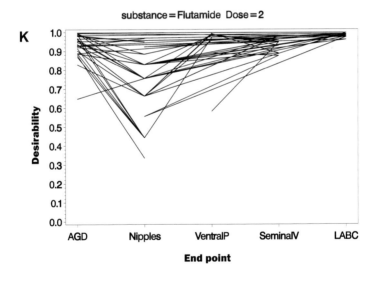

substance = Flutamide Dose = 2

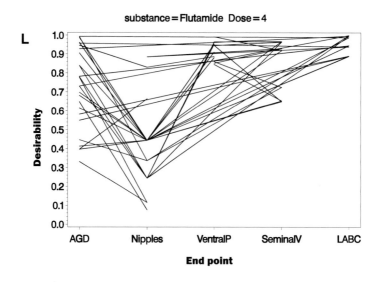

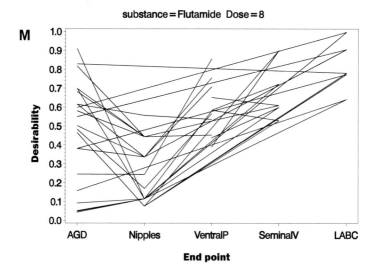

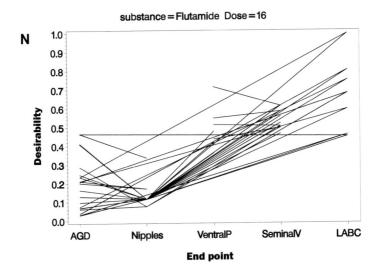

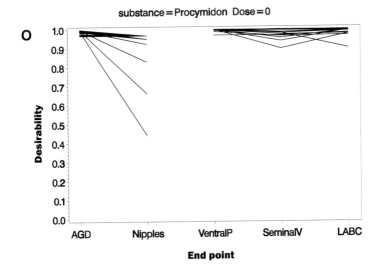

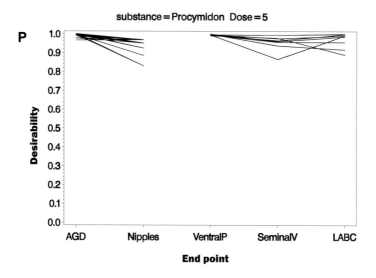

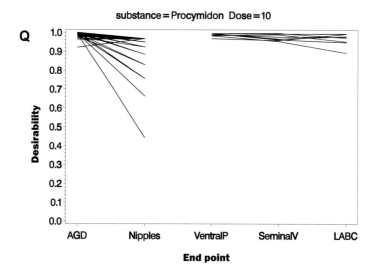

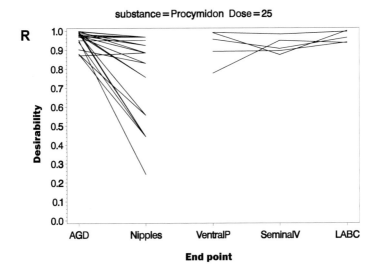

substance = Procymidon Dose = 25

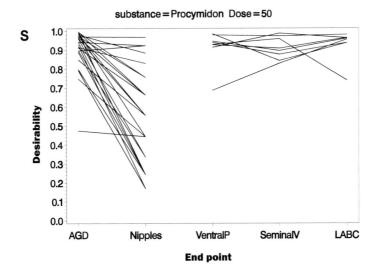

substance = Procymidon Dose = 50

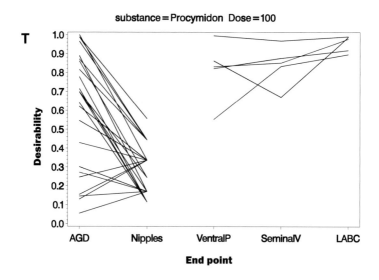

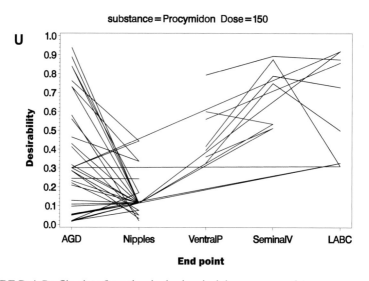

FIGURE D-4 Profile plots from the single chemical dose-response data.

REFERENCES

Casey, M., C. Gennings, W.H. Carter, V.C. Moser, and J.E. Simmons. 2004. Detecting interaction(s) and assessing the impact of component subsets in a chemical mixture using fixed-ratio mixture ray designs. JABES 9(3):339-361.

Coffey, J.T., C. Gennings, and V.M. Moser. 2007. The simultaneous analysis of discrete and continuous outcomes in a dose-response study: Using desirability functions. Regul. Toxicol. Pharmacol. 48(1):51-58.

Derringer, G. 1994. A balancing act: Optimizing a product's properties. Quality Progress 27(June):51-58.

Derringer, G., and R. Suich. 1980. Simultaneous optimization of several response variables. J. Qual. Technol. 12:214-219.

Ellis, R., C, Gennings, J. Benson, and B. Tibbetts. 2008. Validation of a Morbidity Score in a Study of Botulism Toxin A. The Toxicologist 102(S1):240[Abstract 1165].

EPA (U.S. Environmental Protection Agency). 2002. A Review of the Reference Dose and Reference Concentration Processes. Final report. EPA/630/P-02/002F. Risk Assessment Forum, U.S. Environmental Protection Agency, Washington, DC. December 2002 [online]. Available: http://cfpub.epa.gov/ncea/cfm/recordisplay.cfm?deid=55365 [accessed Oct. 9, 2008].

EPA (U.S. Environmental Protection Agency). 2005. Guidelines for Carcinogen Risk Assessment. EPA/630/P-03/001F. Risk Assessment Forum, U.S. Environmental Protection Agency, Washington, DC. March 2005 [online]. Available: http://cf pub.epa.gov/ncea/cfm/recordisplay.cfm?deid=116283 [accessed Oct. 9, 2008].

Faes, C., H. Geys, M. Aerts, G. Molenberghs, and P.J. Catalano. 2004. Modeling combined continuous and ordinal outcomes in a clustered setting. JABES 9(4):515-530.

Geys, H., G. Molenberghs, and L.M. Ryan. 1999. Pseudolikelihood modeling of multivariate outcomes in developmental toxicology. J. Am. Stat. Assoc. 94(447):734-745.

Geys, H., M.M. Regan, P.J. Catalano, and G. Molenberghs. 2001. Two latent variable risk assessment approach for mixed continuous and discrete outcomes from developmental toxicity data. JABES 6(3):340-355.

Harrington, E.C., Jr. 1965. The desirability function. Ind. Qual. Control 21(10):494-498.

Hass, U., M. Scholze, S. Christiansen, M. Dalgaard, A.M. Vinggaard, M. Axelstad, S.B. Metzdorff, and A. Kortenkamp. 2007. Combined exposure to anti-androgens exacerbates disruption of sexual differentiation in the rat. Environ. Health Perspect.115(S1):122-128.

McDaniel, K.L., and V.C. Moser. 1993. Utililty of a neurobehavioral screening battery for differentiating the effects of two pyrethroids, permethrin and cypermethrin. Neurotoxicol. Teratol. 15(2):71-83.

Metzdorff, S.B., M. Kalgaard, S. Christiansen, M. Axelstad, U. Hass, M.K. Kiersgaard, M Scholze, A. Kortenkamp, and A.M. Vinggaard. 2007. Dysgenesis and histological changes of genitals and perturbations of gene expression in male rats after in utero exposure to antiandrogen mixtures. Toxicol. Sci. 98(1):87-98.

Moser, V.C. 1991. Applications of a neurobehavioral screening battery. Int. J. Toxicol. 10(6):661-669.

Moser, V.C., B.M. Cheek, and R.C. MacPhail. 1995. A multidisciplinary approach to toxicological screening. III. Neurobehavioral toxicity. J. Toxicol. Environ. Health 45(2):173-210.

Moser, V.C., G.C. Becking, V. Cuomo, E. Frantík, B.M. Kulig, R.C. MacPhail, H.A. Tilson, G. Winneke, W.S. Brightwell, M.A. De Salvia, M.W. Gill, G.C. Haggerty, M. Hornychová, J. Lammers, J.J. Larsen, K.L. McDaniel, B.K. Nelson, and G. Ostergaard. 1997. The IPCS collaborative study on neurobehavioral screening methods: V. Results of chemical testing. Neurotoxicology 18(4):969-1056.

Regan, M.M., and P.J. Catalano. 1999. Bivariate dose-response modeling and risk estimation in developmental toxicology. JABES 4(3):217-237.

Sammel, M.D., L.M. Ryan, and J.M. Legler. 1997. Latent variable models for mixed discrete and continuous outcomes. J. Roy. Stat. Soc. B 59(3):667-678.

Shih, M., C. Gennings, V.M. Chinchilli, and W.H. Carter Jr. 2003. Titrating and evaluating multi-drug regimens within subjects. Stat. Med. 22(14):2257-2279.

Wu, F.C. 2005. Optimization of correlated multiple quality characteristics using desirability function. Qual. Eng. 17(1):119-126.